The New Arthritis Cure

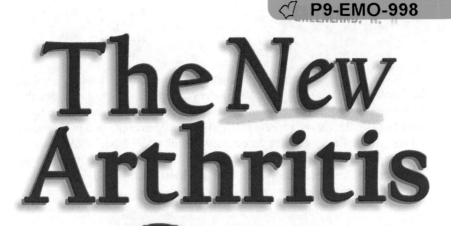

Eliminate Arthritis and Fibromyalgia Pain Permanently

Dr. Bruce Fife

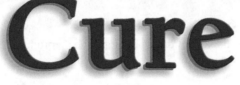

Piccadilly Books, Ltd.
Colorado Springs, CO

Every effort has been made to ensure that the information contained in this book is complete and accurate. However, neither the publisher nor the author is engaged in rendering professional advice or services to the individual reader. The ideas, procedures, and suggestions contained in this book are not intended as a substitute for consulting with your physician. All matters regarding your health require medical supervision. Neither the author nor the publisher shall be liable or responsible for any loss of damage allegedly arising from any information or suggestion in this book.

Piccadilly Books, Ltd.
P.O. Box 25203
Colorado Springs, CO 80936, USA
info@piccadillybooks.com
www.piccadillybooks.com

Library of Congress Cataloging-in-Publication Data
Fife, Bruce, 1952-
    The new arthritis cure: eliminate arthritis and fibromyalgia pain permanently / by Bruce Fife.
        p. cm.
    Includes bibliographical references and index.
    ISBN 978-0-941599-82-5 (pbk.)
    1. Arthritis--Alternative treatment. 2. Fibromyalgia--Alternative treatment. 3. Naturopathy. I. Title.
    RC933.F495 2009
    616.7'2206--dc22
                                                2009016792
Published in the USA

Table of Contents

Chapter 1

There Is A Cure
for Arthritis

"Amazing results!" exclaims Barbara. "I have had chronic pain for 10 years." After following the program in this book for only four weeks, she says, "Here are the results I have noticed so far. *Reversed* documented nerve impingement and foot drop (inability to heel walk). *Reversed* documented osteoarthritis of my spine and knees. *Avoided* my fifth spine surgery and threatened second fusion. *Restored* my ability to exercise. I am able to walk down a flight of stairs *without* pain, limping or gimping. I can also walk two miles without knee pain!...My prior problems were well documented with MRI and PET scans that showed nerve impingement, lack of ankle reflex and foot drop, inability to resist downward pressure on my great toe and foot. Then only four weeks later, I had a perfectly normal EMG; I could heel walk; and I had a normal ankle reflex and good toe, foot, and ankle strength. The fact that this was so well documented, my doctors were completely amazed and interested. The doctor who did my EMG wanted the name of your book, as did my surgeon."

Sylvia had a similar experience. She states, "I have been suffering from arthritis in the knees for the last 10 years and pain in the lower back for the last two decades. I have tried several allopathic medicines and got temporary relief. I started doing [your program] and observed miraculous changes happening. Within five days my arthritis in the knees and lower back pain are *completely* cured. It is just unbelievable!"

5

"I started a few months ago," says Tracy. "Arthritis in my fingers is gone and has never returned. Several chronic pains other than my fingers have also gone away."

Do you suffer from osteoarthritis, rheumatoid arthritis, gout, or fibromyalgia? If so, this book may have the solution you have been looking for.

The title of this book, *The New Arthritis Cure*, makes a rather bold statement since it promises to "cure" a disease that medical science has yet to fully understand, let alone cure. But the title is completely accurate. The information in this book can bring about a complete cure or at least significant improvement for most forms of arthritis. The word *New* is included in the title to indicate that much of the information discussed in this book is completely new to most people and even to many doctors. Another reason to add *New* to the title is because another book, *The Arthritis Cure*, already exists; a distinction needed to be made between the two. This other book makes no mention of the underlying cause and only offers dietary supplements as a solution. In contrast, the book you are now reading outlines a program that will bring about significant relief to the vast majority of arthritis and fibromyalgia sufferers. How can I make such a bold statement when no other book or treatment comes close? The reason is that most physicians believe arthritis to be incurable. They do not understand the cause, therefore, they have no idea where to look for the cure.

In this book, you will learn exactly what causes arthritis and what you can do to cure it. This method works because it addresses the root of the problem, not the symptoms. Once the causative factors are resolved, the disease goes away! It is that simple.

There are many methods for treating arthritis, both medically and alternatively. In conventional medicine, treatment is focused on relieving the symptoms with anti-inflammatory medications and painkillers. This approach does nothing to fix the problem; it merely masks the symptoms while the disease progresses and worsens. In time, the patient becomes crippled or is in need of invasive surgery—an unfortunate and drastic action to a problem that has a simple solution.

Alternative or natural remedies take a different approach. The basic philosophy is that if you improve the health of the entire individual,

6

then the body's own recuperative powers can bring about healing. While this philosophy is accurate, the approach to improving health can take on various forms with varying degrees of success. Eating a healthy diet is an essential element in achieving better health. But what is a healthy diet? Some would say a low-fat vegetarian diet, while others will claim a moderate-fat low-carbohydrate diet is the way to go. And still others may proclaim the virtues of the macrobiotic diet, blood type diet, or any number of diets that happen to be popular at the time. So which diet do you choose?

Even if you are lucky enough to choose a diet that truly promotes better health, there is no guarantee that it alone can bring about a cure. In cases where a degenerative disease, such as arthritis, has become chronic, diet alone is often not enough to reverse all the damage in a reasonable amount of time and bring about complete recovery. Something more is needed to stimulate repair and speed healing.

There are numerous natural remedies that are said to aid those with arthritis, such as eating fresh garlic or drinking solutions of vinegar and honey. For some people, these home remedies seem to work, or at least ease the symptoms. If they do work, however, they don't bring lasting relief because the underlying cause is not addressed. These remedies must be used daily to prevent symptoms from recurring.

Detoxification and fasting methods are also used. Extended fasts in which only water or juice are consumed have long been known to be effective in reducing symptoms associated with arthritis. This has been well documented in published medical studies. However, after the fast is over and normal eating resumes, arthritis comes roaring right back. Only when the fast is followed by a diet composed predominately of natural, fresh foods (as opposed to refined grains, sweets, and packaged foods) is there any hope of keeping arthritis at bay. But the diet must be maintained for life, or the disease is likely to return.

Since arthritis can be kept in check by a strict diet, some investigators have proposed that arthritis occurs as a result of an allergic reaction. Something in the diet causes the disease. This has never been proven, and as you will see in this book, allergies are not the cause. Although food allergies can encourage or exacerbate arthritis, they do so by interfering with and depressing immune function.

7

The only way to achieve a permanent cure for arthritis is to address the underlying cause. Surprisingly, science has known the cause for over a century. Since the early part of the twentieth century, researchers have observed a strong association between arthritis and infection. Microorganisms invade the joint tissue causing inflammation, swelling, damage, and pain—the classic symptoms of arthritis. They alter blood chemistry, producing all the markers doctors use to categorize the various forms of arthritis.

Researchers have identified dozens of bacteria, viruses, and fungi that can and do invade joint tissues and cause arthritis. These organisms have been found in the blood and joint tissues of people suffering from all the major forms of arthritis, including osteoarthritis, rheumatoid arthritis, and gout. There is even a link between infection and fibromyalgia.

It is well known that acute infections such as Lyme disease, gonorrhea, salmonella, pneumonia, and the like can and often do cause arthritis. Arthritis develops during or soon after the onset of the disease. Often, after the systemic infection is brought under control and health is restored to "normal," arthritis continues and becomes chronic—a residual effect of the infection. What hasn't been as evident, until now, is that less dramatic or less noticeable infections can also be the genesis of chronic arthritis. Urinary tract infections, yeast (candida) infections, the flu, and even periodontal (dental) infections can trigger the processes that lead to arthritis.

The fact that infection is a major cause of arthritis is not new or even really controversial. The real issue here is how to treat it. Up till now, treatment has consisted almost entirely of anti-inflammatory drugs and painkillers, which do absolutely nothing to stop the disease. Antibiotics have also been used with varying degrees of success. But still, they aren't the answer, as you will soon discover.

Knowing the cause allows us to formulate a plan of action, an "Arthritis Battle Plan," so to speak, to stop the progression of the disease and to encourage regeneration and recovery. Yes, there is a cure for arthritis. In this book you will see the evidence for the infection connection and discover how and why infections influence joint health. More importantly, you will be shown the steps you must take in order to stop the disease process and regain your health.

Chapter 2

The Many Faces of Arthritis

Most doctors shrug their shoulders and accept the inevitable when treating patients with arthritis, prescribing nothing more than painkillers and anti-inflammatory drugs.

Medical textbooks say there is no cure for most forms of arthritis. Medical treatment focuses on easing the symptoms, not on curing the affliction. The problem doctors face in treating arthritis is that, although there are many theories, they really don't know what causes it. If they don't know the cause, then they don't know where to look for the cure. So the question is: Can arthritis be cured? The answer is a resounding *yes!* Arthritis can be cured. Science has identified the cause and knows the cure. These facts aren't hidden or unknown, though they aren't widely publicized, either. Up to now, most of those in the medical establishment have turned a deaf ear to the exciting studies that are unlocking the secrets of arthritis.

Doctors, in general, are overly cautious and extraordinarily slow at recognizing and accepting new theories that contrast with established dogma or cherished beliefs. Many doctors have built careers based on these beliefs, and the thought of abandoning them in favor of new theories is met with stiff resistance. Dramatic changes in medical thought often take decades and even a generation or two before they are generally accepted. Acceptance usually happens one doctor at a time until one day the new concept is embraced by everyone as being obvious.

Right now, there is a cure for arthritis, or at least for most forms of it. You don't have to wait decades or an entire generation for the medical community to catch up. You can start right now and cure yourself in a matter of weeks or months. Nothing in this program is harmful, painful, or expensive, so you aren't losing anything by trying it. Only in severe cases will more extensive work be needed to accomplish a permanent cure. So what do you have to lose? Only your pain and immobility.

What's In the Joint?

Joints are formed where two bones meet. All of your bones, except for one (the hyoid bone in your neck), form joints with other bones. Joints hold your bones together and allow your body to move. The adult human body has 206 bones with over 230 *moveable* joints (all of which are potential sites for arthritis). There are three basic types of joints: *fixed, slightly moveable,* and *freely moveable.* Fixed joints, like the sutures in your skull, allow essentially no movement. Slightly moveable joints allow for only a small amount of movement. The vertebrae are connected by this type of joint and so are the teeth. Although appearing to be immovable, the teeth move just enough for us to sense how hard we are biting and whether we have food stuck between them. Freely movable joints act as hinges, levers, and pivots and allow us to bend, stand, run, walk, jump, kneel, grasp, pull and otherwise perform the thousands of movements we do each day. Most of the joints in the body are moveable.

Each joint is a complex unit of bone, cartilage, ligament, and other structures that make movement possible. Surrounding the entire joint is the *joint capsule.* This capsule is made of tough, fibrous, connective tissue and is firmly attached to the shaft of each bone to provide a covering over the joint. Inside this capsule is the *synovial membrane.* This membrane is filled with a slippery liquid called *synovial fluid,* which acts as a lubricant for the joint. Ligaments are cordlike structures made of the same strong connective tissue as the joint capsule and lash the two bones together. The bones are capped with a layer of cartilage (called *articular cartilage*) which acts as a shock absorber and protective pad to keep the bones from coming into direct contact

10

with each other. The synovial fluid lubricates the junction between the cartilage of each bone end to allow for easier movement (see diagram on page 13).

A Look at Arthritis

Arthritis afflicts countless millions of people worldwide, including one in five adults in the United States. It is the most widespread crippling disease in America. In this country over 50 percent of adults 65 years of age or older have been diagnosed with the disease. An estimated 294,000 (1 in every 250) children under the age of 18 have some form of it.

Arthritis is also called *degenerative joint disease*. The word *arthritis* means "joint inflammation." Arthritis is not a single disease but a group of diseases whose common characteristics include pain, inflammation, and limited movement of the joints. There are more than 100 diseases that affect the joints. The two most common types of arthritis are osteoarthritis and rheumatoid arthritis.

The term *arthritis* is widely misused and is frequently applied to vague aches and pains in almost any part of the body. Therefore, a diagnosis must be made by a physician to accurately identify the disease. Arthritis can afflict any joint but is most common in the knees, wrists, elbows, fingers, toes, hips, and shoulders. The neck and back also may become arthritic. If you do feel pain in a joint, however, it may not always indicate arthritis, because other parts, such as ligaments and tendons, also make up the structure of the joint.

Arthritis may involve one joint or many. Symptoms of chronic arthritis are pain, swelling, stiffness, and deformity in one or more joints. The signs may appear suddenly or come on gradually. Victims feel aches and pains that vary from a sharp, burning sensation to grinding pain. Moving the affected joint usually hurts, although sometimes it is only stiff.

Often, pain increases with exposure to cold and dampness. Other factors that influence the condition include poor diet, lack of exercise, overweight, infections, and injury to a joint or constant strain upon it. The most common forms of arthritis are described briefly below. As you read the descriptions for each one, look for the similarities among

11

them. Here you will discover the underlying cause of all the major forms of arthritis.

Osteoarthritis

Osteoarthritis is by far the most common form of arthritis comprising approximately 80 percent of all cases. If you have arthritis, it is most likely osteoarthritis. The risk of developing osteoarthritis increases with age. It affects about 2 percent of the population under the age of 45, 30 percent between the ages of 45 and 64, and 50 to 85 percent of those over the age of 65, many of which are undiagnosed.

Osteoarthritis is frequently referred to as a *noninflammatory* joint disease because it does not always involve inflammation. Although inflammation may be present and anti-inflammatory drugs are often prescribed, it is not as pronounced as it is in other forms of arthritis.

Osteoarthritis is a degenerative condition and has often been considered a disease of old age. It is characterized by the wearing away or degeneration of the cartilage on the ends of the bone. One end of a bone then rubs against another, causing stiffness and sometimes pain. The disease most often attacks the joints that carry weight or undergo a great deal of wear and tear, such as the knees, hips, lower spine, toes, and fingers.

It is often referred to as "wear and tear" arthritis because those joints that undergo the most stress or trauma are the first to experience symptoms. Doctors often tell us that it is a consequence of aging and that it is both unavoidable and incurable.

While the risk of developing osteoarthritis increases with age, it is not a normal part of the aging process and is not caused simply by age. Many people live long lives without ever developing the condition. We now know that there are striking differences between joints and cartilage that are affected by osteoarthritis and those that have simply aged normally.[1] The deterioration that happens as a normal process of aging occurs uniformly on all joints; in osteoarthritis it occurs on weight-bearing surfaces. Aging shows minimal physical and chemical change in cartilage and bone. In osteoarthritis there are significant physical, chemical, and degenerative changes in the cartilage and bone.

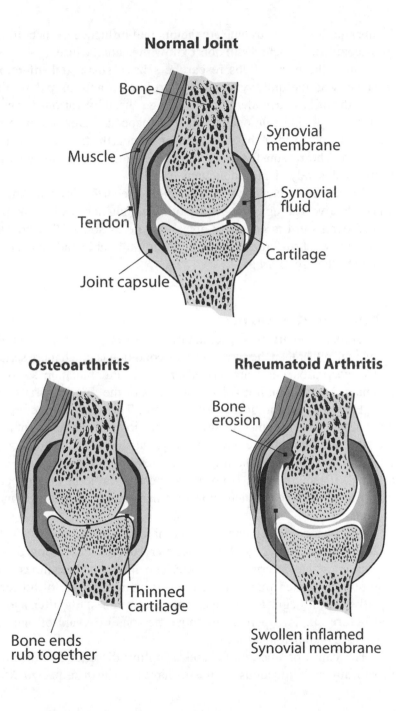

Normal Joint

Bone

Synovial membrane

Muscle

Synovial fluid

Tendon

Cartilage

Joint capsule

Osteoarthritis

Rheumatoid Arthritis

Bone erosion

Thinned cartilage

Bone ends rub together

Swollen inflamed Synovial membrane

While age, stress, and trauma are factors that influence the occurrence of osteoarthritis, doctors still don't know the actual cause.

Since the early 1900s researchers have suspected infectious organisms as the underlying cause.[2] In human and animal studies, osteoarthritis has been identified as being caused by various forms of bacteria, including salmonella and streptococcus.[3] Doctors have not yet accepted the idea that all cases of osteoarthritis are caused by infection. The reason for this is that infectious organisms have not been conclusively identified in many cases.

Osteoarthritis can become crippling. Osteoarthritis of the knee is one of the five leading causes of disability among non-institutionalized adults; even so, it is generally not as severe as some other arthritic disorders. Most sufferers find the condition tolerable and manage the pain with the use of drugs.

Rheumatoid Arthritis

Unlike osteoarthritis, rheumatoid arthritis affects the synovial membrane rather than the cartilage. This condition is much more serious than osteoarthritis. It is characterized by chronic inflammation, swelling, and pain. Most often, it involves the joints of the fingers, wrists, and feet. However, any joint may be affected. The synovial membrane that lines the joint becomes inflamed, and the joint swells up. Eventually, the surrounding cartilage is worn away, causing the joint to become exceedingly painful and hard to move. Neighboring muscles are also affected. If the condition is not treated early, the joint may become immovable. Careful treatment, however, may prevent disability in most persons.

The observed incidence of rheumatoid arthritis in the United States ranges from 42 to 68 persons per 100,000 depending on the definition used to describe the disease. The disease is three times more common in women than it is in men. It afflicts people of all races equally. It can begin at any age, but most often starts after age 40 and before 60. Two percent of those persons 60 years of age and older have rheumatoid arthritis.

The cause of this painful and crippling disorder is still under debate, although infectious organisms have long been suspected. Most doctors believe it to be an autoimmune disorder, in which the body's immune system attacks itself. Antibodies that the body produces to protect itself from infection become turncoats and attack joint tissue as well as other organs in the body.

Because it can affect multiple organs, rheumatoid arthritis is referred to as a systemic illness and is sometimes referred to as rheumatoid disease or rheumatism. Patients can experience long periods without symptoms. Typically, however, rheumatoid arthritis is a progressive illness that has the potential to cause joint destruction and disability.

Gout and Pseudogout

Have you ever awakened in the middle of the night feeling like your big toe is on fire? It's hot, tender, and swollen, with shooting pain at the slightest touch? If you have, then you may have been experiencing an acute attack of gout. Gout is a form of arthritis that is characterized by sudden, severe attacks of pain, redness, and tenderness in the joints.

Gouty arthritis is considered a metabolic condition in which uric acid, a nitrogenous waste from the breakdown of purine, increases in the blood. Excess uric acid accumulates as sodium urate crystals in joints and other tissues. Pseudogout is a very similar condition, but instead of sodium urate, the crystals are composed predominately of calcium.

Historically, gout has been associated with gluttony. It was considered a disease of royalty who feasted heavily on purine-rich foods such as meat and wine. Charlemagne and King Henry VIII are among those who suffered from gout. Today gout sufferers are often encouraged to reduce their meat and alcohol consumption in the belief that it might forestall attacks.

Although excess alcohol or meat consumption may increase the chances of suffering an acute attack of gout, neither one actually causes the disease. Most people with gout do not produce more than the normal amount of uric acid (a byproduct of protein metabolism). Instead, they are unable to completely excrete the uric acid they produce. The kidneys are responsible for approximately one third of uric acid excretion, with the gut responsible for the rest. Many people with high levels of uric acid have kidney troubles. About 20 percent of patients with gout also develop kidney stones.[4-5]

Complications associated with kidney stones include obstruction in the urinary tract and infection. If left untreated, gout can lead to progressive kidney disease. Gout is often complicated by other medical conditions such as high blood pressure. This causes more crystals to be deposited in joints, causing additional attacks.

Gout is the most common type of inflammatory arthritis among men. Lifetime prevalence estimates are 2.6 percent overall for those over 20 years of age, with a low of 400 per 100,000 in adults aged 20 to 29 years and a peak of 8,000 per 100,000 in adults aged 70 to 79 years. Gout is reported more often in men than in women overall, but prevalence increases with age for both, especially for postmenopausal women.

The shooting pain and inflammation characteristic of gout attacks are believed to be triggered by the sharp crystals piercing tender joint tissues. Movement can cause excruciating pain. Attacks occur suddenly, can last for days or weeks, and then suddenly disappear, only to resurface a few months or a year later. Gout usually affects only one joint at a time.

Treatment for gout consists of nonsteroidal anti-inflammatory drugs (NSAIDs) for pain and inflammation, abstinence from alcohol, restriction of protein-rich foods, and possibly medications to reduce uric acid production or increase its excretion. Dietary restrictions may or may not help. Restriction of milk or calcium-rich foods seems to have no effect on pseudogout, which is associated with calcium crystals.

Gout is notorious for producing symptoms indicating the presence of an acute infection and is often "misdiagnosed" as such. It displays the appearance of a systemic infection that has localized in the joints. Fever, redness, hot joints, and elevated white blood cell count are characteristic of gout attacks. The only way for doctors to identify it is to remove a sample of synovial fluid and test for the presence of crystals and bacteria. If crystals are present it is diagnosed as gout; if bacteria is present it is diagnosed as infectious arthritis (see Infectious Arthritis section below).

The common belief that the presence of "needle-sharp" crystals are the cause of gout attacks is highly improbable. These crystals grow very slowly, taking years to develop. Why, all of a sudden, in the middle of the night when the joints aren't even being used, would the edges of the crystals start to stab the joints and cause pain, inflammation, and swelling? If irritating crystals grew there over time, the pain would develop gradually, increasing in intensity day by day. And the symptoms wouldn't just suddenly end all by themselves, but would continue as long as the crystals were present. Gout crystals don't instantaneously disappear; they remain for life unless something drastic happens that changes the body's chemistry and causes them to dissolve.

Gout attacks come and go for no apparent reason. The crystals are not the cause but are a symptom, just like kidney stones don't cause kidney disease; they are a symptom of a malfunctioning kidney. So what causes gout?

Although gout produces all the signs of an acute infection, it isn't believed to be caused by an infection because of the absence of bacteria in the synovial fluid and the failure of gout to respond to antibiotic treatment. It is very possible that a virus could be the cause. Viruses can avoid detection by typical lab tests and are not affected by antibiotics. This also explains the unusual nature of gout attacks coming and going periodically for no apparent reason. The same thing occurs with other viral infections. Herpes, for example, will remain dormant for months or years and then suddenly flare up as a cold sore on the lips. It causes an acute infection accompanied by redness and blistering for a few days and then fades away, only to return another day. At this time, like most other forms of arthritis, doctors really don't know what causes gout.

Juvenile Arthritis

Juvenile arthritis is a form of rheumatoid arthritis that occurs in children. It involves at least six weeks of persistent arthritis in a child younger than 16 years with no other type of childhood arthritis. Girls are more commonly affected than boys. It usually clears up after a few years, but about 40 to 45 percent have the active disease for over 10 years. The peak age of onset is one to six years of age and may stunt growth and leave the child with permanent deformities.

In some cases, symptoms can be systemic (*systemic juvenile rheumatoid arthritis,* also known as Still's disease). These symptoms can easily be mistaken for the flu or for food poisoning. They may involve a fever of 102 degrees F (39 C) or more, that may disappear and reappear the next day, accompanied by shaking chills, swollen lymph nodes, and a faint salmon-colored skin rash. Appetite may be poor, with weight loss, stomach pain, severe anemia, sore throat, and a high white blood cell count. These symptoms may last for weeks or even months. Arthritis, with joint swelling, often occurs after the rash and fevers have been present for some time.

A form of juvenile arthritis called *polyarticular juvenile rheumatoid arthritis* affects several joints (five or more). It often strikes symmetrically, affecting the same joint on both sides of the body. In some cases, the patient may also experience a slight fever and eye inflammation. It often develops into *ankylosing spondylitis* (see below) as the child approaches adulthood.

Ankylosing Spondylitis

Ankylosing spondylitis (AS) is a chronic, painful, inflammatory arthritis primarily affecting the spine and sacroiliac joints (the joints where the lower spine meets the pelvis). It usually begins in the lower back and later affects the middle and upper back. It may spread to other joints and often affects the hips. The tendons and ligaments that make it possible to move the back become inflamed. In response, the vertebrae grow into each other and fuse together. The spine can end up looking something like a bamboo pole, bending forward under the weight of the head. If you have ever seen an elderly person walking bent over as though he were looking at this feet, you have probably witnessed the late stages of AS.

The disease typically begins at a relatively young age, 18 to 30 years. Pain is often severe on rest, and improves with physical activity. Men are affected more than women by a ratio of about 3:1. In 40 percent of cases, it is associated with eye pain and sensitivity to light; another common symptom is generalized fatigue. When the condition occurs before the age of 18, it is likely to cause pain and swelling of large limb joints, particularly the knees.

18

Most doctors don't really know what causes AS, but the overwhelming evidence is that it is caused by a combination of genetic susceptibility and infection. The infection apparently triggers the onset of the disease in genetically susceptible individuals. It is often associated with gastrointestinal infections and Crohn's disease. The belief is that intestinal bacteria enter the bloodstream, generally through an ulcer in the gastrointestinal tract, initiating AS. Organisms that have been associated with AS include campylobacter, clostridium, salmonella, shigella, yersinia, bacteroides, and especially the bacterium *Klebsiella pneumoniae*.[6-10] The gene that is associated with AS susceptibility is called HLA-B27. Studies show that rats bred with this gene and kept in a sterile environment do not develop AS unless they are infected with one of these organisms. Unfortunately, antibiotics have not proven very successful in controlling this disease.

Approximately 90 percent of those who develop AS have the gene HLA-B27; this is why it is believed to be a genetic disorder. However, what about the 10 percent who don't have the gene but still have the disease? Why did they get the disease? Genetics doesn't appear to be the complete answer.

Reactive Arthritis

Reactive arthritis, formerly called Reiter's syndrome, shares many features with ankylosing spondylitis. Reactive arthritis is a chronic form of arthritis with three distinguishing features: inflamed joints, inflammation of the eyes, and inflammation of the genital, urinary or gastrointestinal systems. This form of arthritis is called "reactive" arthritis because the immune system is "reacting" to the presence of a bacterial infection in the genital, urinary, or gastrointestinal system.

Reactive arthritis is considered a systemic rheumatic disease. This means it can affect organs other than the joints, causing inflammation in tissues such as the eyes, mouth, skin, kidneys, heart, and lungs.

Like AS, reactive arthritis is believed to be caused by the combination of genetics and infection. The same gene seen in those with AS, HLA-B27, appears to be common in reactive arthritis patients as well. Exposure to certain infections is required to trigger the onset of the disease. Reactive arthritis can occur after venereal infections. The most common bacterium that has been associated with this post-

19

venereal form of reactive arthritis is *Chlamydia trachomatis*. A bout of food poisoning or a gastrointestinal or urinary tract infection may also precede the disease.[11] Typically, symptoms develop one to three weeks after the onset of the bacterial infection. The interaction between the infecting organism and the host is not fully understood. Bacterial cultures of synovial fluid are generally negative, which leads to the belief that reactive arthritis is an autoimmune disease caused by an over-stimulated immune response that, for some unknown reason, becomes chronic. Treatment consists of painkillers, NSAIDs, and immune system suppressants.

Psoriatic Arthritis

Psoriatic arthritis is a chronic disease characterized by inflammation of the skin (psoriasis) and the joints. Psoriasis is a common skin condition affecting 2 percent of the Caucasian population in the United States. It is characterized by patchy, raised, red areas of skin inflammation with scaling. Psoriasis often affects the ends of the elbows and knees, the scalp, the navel, and around the genitalia. Approximately 10 percent of patients with psoriasis also develop psoriatic arthritis.

Psoriatic arthritis generally occurs sometime after the age of 40. Male and females are affected equally. Skin outbreak and joint pain usually appear separately with the skin condition preceding the joint pain in about 80 percent of patients. Up to 15 percent of patients develop arthritis prior to the rash. Diagnosis of psoriatic arthritis can be difficult if the arthritis precedes the psoriasis by many years. In fact, patients can have arthritis for 20 years or more before psoriasis appears. Conversely, patients can have psoriasis for many years prior to developing arthritis.

In most patients, psoriasis precedes arthritis by months or years. The arthritis frequently involves the knees, ankles, and joints in the feet, but can also affect the spine and lower back. Inflammation in the fingers or toes can cause swelling of the entire digit, giving them the appearance of sausages. Joint stiffness is common and is typically worse early in the morning.

Psoriatic arthritis is a systemic disease that can cause inflammation in other areas of the body besides the joints, such as the eyes, heart, lungs, and kidneys. Psoriatic arthritis shares many features with other forms of arthritis such as ankylosing spondylitis and reactive arthritis.

The cause is currently unknown, but like ankylosing spondylitis, it is believed to be a combination of genetics and infection. Patients with psoriatic arthritis have the HLA-B27 gene about 50 percent of the time. Doctors assume that there must be other defective genes responsible for the other 50 percent.

Fibromyalgia

Your joints are stiff, you hurt all over, you have difficulty sleeping, and you feel exhausted all the time. Lab tests show nothing amiss and your doctor cannot find anything specifically wrong with you. Does this sound familiar? If so, you may have fibromyalgia.

The term *fibromyalgia* comes from the combination of the Latin word *fibro* (fiber) and Greek words *myo* (muscle) and *algos* (pain), meaning muscle and connective tissue pain.

Fibromyalgia is considered an arthritis-related condition. However, technically, it is not a form of arthritis because it does not cause damage or inflammation in the joints, muscles, or other tissues. Fibromyalgia can, like arthritis, cause significant pain. It is often associated with joint stiffness and pain in nearby areas. It is included here because fibromyalgia appears to have an origin similar to arthritis, and sufferers respond well to the techniques discussed in this book.

This disorder is characterized by chronic widespread pain in the muscles, ligaments, and tendons and a heightened and painful response to gentle touch. It can involve a wide range of other symptoms, including moderate-to-severe fatigue, insomnia, joint stiffness, numbness or needlelike tingling of the skin, muscle aches, prolonged muscle spasms, muscle weakness, nerve pain, abdominal pain, bloating, nausea, constipation alternating with diarrhea, headaches, jaw and facial tenderness, difficulty concentrating on and performing simple mental tasks, increase in urinary urgency or frequency, reduced tolerance for exercise, a feeling of swelling (without actual swelling)

21

in the hands and feet, painful menstrual periods, dizziness, and sensitivity to odors, noise, bright lights, medications, certain foods, and cold. Those suffering from this condition don't usually experience all of these symptoms but may encounter any combination of them.

For many years, fibromyalgia was not officially recognized as a medical condition. The reason for this is that laboratory tests don't show any abnormalities that are characteristic of the condition, and it involves such a variety of symptoms that it is difficult to diagnose. Because of the difficulty in diagnosing this condition, it is often called the *invisible syndrome*. It was often considered a psychological disorder and doctors believed people just thought they felt bad. It wasn't until 1990 that the American College of Rheumatology officially recognized fibromyalgia as a genuine health disorder. Because there are no diagnostic tests, it is referred to as a *syndrome* rather than a disease.

The cause is currently unknown, but several hypotheses have been suggested including genetic predisposition, excessive stress, sleep disturbance, hormone dysfunction, depression, toxin exposure, and infection. The onset of symptoms often occurs after a physical or emotional trauma. Many people diagnosed with fibromyalgia relate that the onset of their symptoms occurred either during or right after a viral infection such as the flu. Certain infections, including hepatitis C, HIV, and Lyme disease, have been associated with the onset of fibromyalgia. There is also evidence for the possible role of vaccinations in triggering the disorder.[12-13]

People with certain rheumatic (connective tissue) diseases, such as rheumatoid arthritis, ankylosing spondylitis, and systemic lupus erythematosus are more likely to also have fibromyalgia, suggesting perhaps a similar cause or path of development. There is no universally accepted cure and standard treatment is aimed at managing symptoms.

(Acute) Infectious Arthritis

Infectious arthritis is also known as septic arthritis. This is a very important, yet underappreciated form of degenerative joint disease and provides a key to understanding the solution to most all other forms of arthritis. It is the only form of arthritis for which doctors know the cause and have a cure. As the name implies, the disease is caused by the invasion of microorganisms, usually bacteria, into the joint from a nearby infected wound or from bacteremia (infection in the bloodstream).

This type of arthritis arises solely from an infection without any known influence from genetics, metabolic disorders, or other complicating factors. It is purely and simply an infection that attacks the joints.

Infectious arthritis occurs in all age groups. In adults, it usually affects the wrists or one of the patient's weight-bearing joints, most often the knee, although about 20 percent of adult patients have symptoms in more than one joint. Multiple joint infections are common in children and typically involve the shoulders, knees, and hips.

Infectious arthritis can be caused by any number of bacteria, viruses, or fungi that find entrance into the joint through the bloodstream. The most common causes are from bacteria, especially *Staphylococcus aureus, Streptococcus pyogenes, Streptococcus viridans,* and *Haemophilus influenzae.* In certain high-risk individuals, other bacteria may cause infectious arthritis. *E. coli* and *Pseudomonas spp.* can cause infectious arthritis in intravenous drug abusers and in the elderly; *Neisseria gonorrhoeae* (bacteria that cause gonorrhea) may cause it in sexually active young adults; and *Salmonella spp.* may cause the disease in young children or in people with sickle cell disease. Older adults are often vulnerable to joint infections caused by gram-negative bacilli, including *salmonella* and *pseudomonas.* Other bacteria that can cause infection include *Mycobacterium tuberculosis,* which causes tuberculosis, and species of the spirochete bacterium that cause Lyme disease and syphilis.

Viruses that can cause infectious arthritis include hepatitis A, B, and C, parvovirus, herpes viruses, HIV (the AIDS virus), HTLV-1, adenovirus, coxsackie viruses, mumps, and ebola. Fungi that cause the disease include histoplasma, coccidiomyces, blastomyces, and candida. Many of the bacteria, viruses, and fungi that cause infectious arthritis are common inhabitants of the human body and inhabit the skin, mouth, or digestive tract. They may be relatively harmless in their respective habitats, but if they get into the bloodstream and end up in the joints they can turn into terrorists.

While joint infection can affect people with no known predisposing risk factors, it more commonly occurs when certain risk situations are present. Risks for the development of infectious arthritis include taking medications that suppress the immune system, intravenous drug abuse, past joint disease or injury (especially those with prosthetic joints), surgery, and underlying medical illnesses including diabetes, alcoholism, cancer, sickle cell anemia, rheumatic diseases (including other forms of arthritis and lupus), and immune deficiency disorders.

Symptoms of acute infectious arthritis include joint pain, swelling, redness, stiffness, and warmth. In many cases, the patient will have fever and chills, although the fever may be only low-grade. Children sometimes develop nausea and vomiting. The joints most commonly affected are the knee, shoulder, wrist, hip, elbow, and the joints of the fingers. Most bacterial and fungal infections affect only one joint or, occasionally, several joints. For example, the bacterium that causes Lyme disease most often infects knee joints. Conococcal bacteria and viruses can infect a few or many joints at the same time. The infection often has a sudden onset, but symptoms sometimes develop over a period of 3 to 14 days.

The diagnosis of infectious arthritis depends on a combination of laboratory testing and physical examination of the affected joint. Infectious arthritis can coexist with other forms of arthritis, rheumatic fever, Lyme disease, or other disorders. A diagnosis is made by taking a sample of synovial fluid from the joint. A white blood cell count is made to see if they are elevated, indicating an immune response to a possible infection. The laboratory can usually grow and identify the infecting bacteria from the joint fluid, unless the person has recently taken antibiotics. However, some bacteria, including those that cause gonorrhea, Lyme disease, syphilis, and a few others, are difficult to recover from joint fluid. If bacteria do grow in culture, the laboratory then tests which antibiotics would be effective.

Treatment includes drainage of the infected synovial fluid from the joint and the immediate administration of antibiotics. Often, intravenous antibiotics are administered in a hospital setting. Intravenous antibiotics are given for about two weeks, or until the inflammation has disappeared. The patient may then take oral antibiotics for up to four weeks.

24

Chapter 3

What Causes Arthritis?

Standard Treatment for Arthritis

Current orthodox medicine has no cure for arthritis. Treatment focuses on managing the symptoms so the patient can better endure the condition. The doctor's advice to patients is often little more than "Take two aspirin and learn to live with it."

Various medications, therapies, and procedures are used in treating different types of arthritis. None of them brings about a cure or permanent relief. While the symptoms may abate temporarily, the disease continues to progress and the joint gradually degenerates. Some of these treatments, particularly non-steroidal anti-inflammatory drugs (NSAIDs) may actually cause more harm than good.[1-2] They may help reduce the inflammation but accelerate bone destruction. Painkillers like aspirin and ibuprofen (Motrin, Advil, Nuprin, etc.) may ease pain but in the long run will actually worsen the condition because they inhibit cartilage formation and accelerate cartilage destruction.

At some point, symptoms may become so severe that surgery is recommended. Various surgical procedures include arthroscopic debridement (removal of damaged cartilage), osteotomy (removing portions of the bone to shorten or change its alignment), or finally, total joint arthroplasty (replacement of both joint surfaces with metal or plastic).

More than a half million Americans per year undergo arthroscopic surgery (debridement and osteotomy) to correct osteoarthritis of the knee, at a cost of $3 billion. Despite this, studies show the surgery to be no better than no surgery at all. Research has shown that fake knee surgery, in which surgeons "pretend" to do surgery while the patient is under light anesthesia produces the same results, indicating that the improvement noted by patients is only psychological.[3] Arthroscopic surgery is also no better than much cheaper, and much less invasive, physical therapy.

Joint replacement surgery is fast becoming a popular form of treatment. In 2004, there were 454,652 total knee replacements performed in the United States, primarily for arthritis. In addition, there were 232,857 total hip replacements, 41,934 shoulder replacements, and 12,055 other joint replacements.

Artificial joints are not permanent fixtures that once they are in place that is the end of it. Prosthetic joints do wear down under normal use, and even the most advanced models have duration limits. As the joint experiences wear and tear, numerous micro-particles are broken off. These tiny foreign substances trigger the immune system, which results in local inflammation and the degeneration of surrounding bone. As the bone disintegrates, the artificial joint becomes lose and wobbly. Most prosthetic joints will last about 10 years, longer if the patient is older and inactive, shorter if the patient is very active. If you are relatively young or happen to live a long time, you will have to have the joint replaced again and again until you die.

The second surgery is much more complicated than the first, and the outcome not nearly as good. Technical problems include the quality of the degenerated bone and the ability to adequately secure the replacement into position. Furthermore, removing the old joint can necessitate more extensive surgery. Together these problems often require much more complex surgical procedures.

Artificial joints also create an ideal location for bacteria to collect, which can lead to infectious arthritis or other infections. Therefore, you will probably need to take antibiotics frequently. For instance, every time you go to the dentist, you will need to take antibiotics to prevent the migration of oral bacteria into the joint. Antibiotics may help stem an acute infection, but they carry risks. They increase the risk of candida and other fungal infections. They kill good bacteria in the gut, which are essential for proper food digestion and nutrient assimilation, thus promoting malnutrition. When antibiotics break down, they form toxins that can damage the liver, kidney, bones, and other organs. So, frequent or long-terms use of antibiotics isn't a good thing.

The Real Cause of Arthritis

Your doctor may tell you, "There is nothing we can do about it and you're going to have to learn to live with it." Such advice offers little hope and instills in the patient a sense of helplessness. Don't be discouraged. There is hope. There *is* a cure for arthritis!

All of the major forms of arthritis, including osteoarthritis, rheumatoid arthritis, and gout are really only variations of one form—infectious arthritis. Many other factors may be involved that can promote or exacerbate the condition, such as diet, allergies, trauma, stress, age, and so forth, but the underlying root cause is infection.

There are only two primary types of arthritis—*acute infectious arthritis* and *chronic infectious arthritis*. Acute infectious arthritis, as described in the previous chapter, occurs suddenly with intensity and is of short duration. It is usually very serious and requires immediate medical attention. It develops as a consequence of microorganisms carried in the blood from an infected wound or ulcer or from an infectious systemic illness.

In contrast, chronic infectious arthritis progresses slowly and lasts a long time. The infection is mild, and symptoms vary from mild to serious. This type of infection stems from another chronic low-grade infection originating elsewhere in the body. The immune system is able to partially control the infection, keeping the symptoms mild in comparison to those of acute infectious arthritis. Clear signs of inflammation may or may not be present, depending on the type of organism involved and the intensity of the infection. The various forms of arthritis arise from different infectious organisms and the severity of the infection.

Infections that migrate to the joints and cause arthritis come from a variety of sources including wounds, insect bites (e.g., mosquito, tick, etc.), inhalation, sexual contact, food poisoning, ulcers, vaccinations, and infected teeth and gums.

Let's take a look at how a seemingly unrelated infection can lead to chronic arthritis. Lyme disease offers a good example.

Lyme disease was first identified in 1975, when mothers living near each other in the city of Lyme, Connecticut made the discovery that about 50 of their children were all diagnosed with rheumatoid arthritis—a rare disease for a child. This unusual clustering of arthritis in a young population led researchers to the identification of the disease. Since that time, Lyme disease has been reported throughout the world.

Lyme disease is caused by spirochetal bacteria from the genus *Borrelia*. Humans can become infected when they are bitten by infected ticks. Since ticks are small and secrete chemicals to prevent itching and bleeding, victims may be completely unaware they have been bitten.

Lyme disease affects different areas of the body in varying degrees as it progresses. From the site of the tick bite, bacteria enter the bloodstream and spread throughout the body. Initially, the disease affects the skin, causing circular, expanding, red rashes. As the bacteria migrate throughout the body, flu-like symptoms such as fever, headache, fatigue, and malaise develop. This stage of the disease may be easily mistaken as the flu. If left untreated, the bacteria find their way to the heart, joints, and nerves, where they cause inflammation and pain. At this stage, the disease has often been misdiagnosed as rheumatoid arthritis, multiple sclerosis, fibromyalgia, chronic fatigue syndrome, lupus, or some other autoimmune disease.

Arthritis caused by Lyme disease involves inflammation, swelling, stiffness, and pain. Usually only one or just a few joints are affected, most commonly the knees.

Borrelia is difficult to identify with standard blood tests, so such tests are generally not helpful, especially in the early stages. A diagnosis is made by a physical exam and by asking if the patient has recently been in regions in which Lyme disease is common.

If diagnosed early, treatment consists of oral antibiotics. In later stages the antibiotics need to be delivered directly into the bloodstream through an IV. Antibiotic therapy may last two to four weeks or more.

After antibiotic treatment, some patients continue to suffer with arthritis and other symptoms, even though there is no evidence of bacteria in the blood. Doctors explain this as an ongoing response by the immune system—an autoimmune reaction. Doctors don't know how to explain it otherwise. However, it would seem reasonable to assume that the bacteria were not completely eradicated. Perhaps, like some other microorganisms, they can find safe haven in certain tissues in the body where antibiotics can't reach them. There they continue to live, being kept from causing a full-blown systemic infection by the immune system while the body continually produces antibodies. Instead of an active acute infection, the condition becomes chronic, but low-grade. Joint pain continues as long as a remnant of the infection remains. The bacterium that causes Lyme disease is only one of the causes of arthritis. Septic or infectious arthritis is known to be caused by a wide array of microorganisms.[4-8]

Let's look at another example. This is an actual case reported in 2008. A 75-year-old man went to the dentist to have an infected tooth pulled. Within 48 hours after the extraction of the tooth, his knee became inflamed and swollen. He initially ignored the symptoms, but his condition worsened. After two weeks of struggling with a fever and general malaise, he went to the hospital for treatment. Doctors diagnosed his condition as an acute systemic infection with septic arthritis. The infection came from oral bacteria released into his bloodstream as a result of pulling the infected tooth.[9] This type of thing isn't unheard of. In fact, to avoid situations like this, dentists often recommend the use of antibiotics whenever invasive dental procedures are performed.[10]

It is of interest to note that blood and synovial fluid samples from this patient initially showed no microorganisms present. Further tests

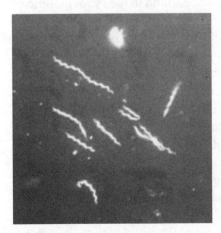

Spirochetes are long, tightly coiled bacteria that look like tiny telephone cords. They include both aerobic and anaerobic species, and both free-living and parasitic forms. Some species thrive in the digestive tract of cows, others prefer the human mouth. Some are the cause of disease, most notably syphilis and Lyme disease.

were run with the same negative results. Doctors knew there must be something there and continued looking. More detailed laboratory analysis eventually revealed the presence of anaerobic bacteria, which shows how difficult it is to find bacteria that don't happen to be among the usual suspects.

Infections from surgery (wounds) as well as ulcers can also cause arthritis.[11-12] Syphilis is known to cause acute infectious arthritis.[13] Another sexually transmitted organism, human papillomavirus (HPV), has been associated with rheumatoid arthritis. HPV is the most prevalent sexually transmitted infection in the world, occurring in up to 75 percent of sexually active women. Although the infection is widespread, few people know they are infected because they seldom have noticeable symptoms. The virus is one of the major causes of cervical cancer as well as arthritis. In one study, researchers found that one out of every three women with rheumatoid arthritis were infected with human papillomavirus.[14]

Food poisoning has often been associated with the onset of chronic arthritis. The bacterium salmonella is a known troublemaker.[15] In one notable instance in 2005, at least 592 individuals in Ontario, Canada developed acute gastroenteritis after consuming bean sprouts contaminated with salmonella. Approximately 46 percent of the victims afterward developed chronic reactive arthritis. Many other studies have suggested that intestinal microbes participate in the genesis of rheumatoid arthritis.[16] Streptococcus, which is a common inhabitant of the skin, mouth, and gastrointestinal tract, is often found in the synovial fluid of arthritic patients.[17]

Although a number of microorganisms have been identified as causing arthritis, one bacterium in particular is even named after the disease. It is called *Mycoplasma arthritidis* or M. arthritidis for short. This organism is routinely used in research to purposely induce chronic and acute arthritis in lab animals. The type of arthritis it induces in animals is virtually identical to human rheumatoid arthritis.[18] When researchers want to induce rheumatoid arthritis in lab animals they inject them with M. arthritidis.

Another microorganism commonly connected with rheumatoid arthritis is the bacterium *Proteus mirabilis*.[19] Proteus is a normal inhabitant of the intestinal tract and is the most frequent cause of urinary tract infections, accounting for more than 80 percent of these infections.

Another inhabitant of the intestinal tract that causes urinary tract infections is E. coli. Both these organisms seem to be involved in the pathogenesis of rheumatoid arthritis. In one study, for instance, out of 76 rheumatoid arthritis patients, 33 percent showed evidence of proteus or E. coli infection in the urinary tract. In 48 control subjects without arthritis, only 4 percent were infected.[20] Blood samples also showed the presence of proteus in the arthritis patients, but in such small numbers that no systemic symptoms were noticeably evident.

"Extensive evidence based on the results of various microbial, immunological, and molecular studies from different parts of the world, shows that a strong link exists between *Proteus mirabilis* microbes and rheumatoid arthritis," says Alan Ebringer, MD, rheumatologist and professor of immunology at Kings College, London. Using a technique called "molecular mimicry" Dr. Ebringer and his team at Kings College demonstrated a clear connection between proteus infection and rheumatoid arthritis. Dr. Ebringer asserts that subclinical, or undetectable, proteus urinary tract infection is a major triggering factor for rheumatoid arthritis.[21] Women are far more likely than men to develop urinary tract infections. This may be one reason why they are also far more likely to develop rheumatoid arthritis.

In addition to proteus, a variety of other bacteria and viruses have also been linked to rheumatoid arthritis.[22-26] Dr. Ebringer recognizes the ineffectiveness of current treatments for rheumatoid arthritis and contends that antimicrobial measures are needed to fight this disease.

Dr. Ebringer and his team at Kings College have also made a connection between ankylosing spondylitis and another intestinal bacterium called *Klebsiella pneumoniae*.[27] Ebringer contends that klebsiella is "the main microbial agent" implicated in triggering this form of arthritis.

Osteoarthritis also appears to result from infection. Researchers can create it in the laboratory. If researchers want to study osteoarthritis in animals, they can induce the disease by injecting candida, a fungus, into the bloodstream. Osteoarthritis develops within days.[28]

Osteoarthritis can occur as a result of a systemic candida infection (candidiasis). An interesting case was reported involving a two-month-old infant girl who was being treated for severe bacterial diarrhea.[77] She was put on antibiotic therapy. The antibiotic killed the infection but also killed the friendly bacteria in her digestive tract. Without

31

competition from this bacteria, candida, which also lives in the digestive tract and is not affected by antibiotics, was allowed to multiply unrestrained. As a consequence, she developed a severe case of candidiasis. The candida attacked her joints, causing osteoarthritis to develope in both of her knees, her left hip, and several other joints. This case is interesting because osteoarthritis is often viewed as a degenerative disease caused by excessive wear and tear, yet here is an example where the disease had clearly not resulted from excessive use since the infant had never walked or even crawled.

People who have had repeated yeast infections or candidiasis usually don't make the connection between the onset of chronic joint pain with a candida overgrowth. Women are the ones most troubled by candida infections and are the ones most affected by osteoarthritis. Candida doesn't appear to be the only cause of osteoarthritis, other organisms are known to be involved as well.[29-31]

Gout, too, is associated with infection.[32-34] Apparently, infection disrupts blood chemistry in some people causing an increase of uric acid levels.

Vaccinations are another source of infection that can affect the joints. Vaccines are preparations which consist of dead or weakened infectious microorganisms. They are injected into the bloodstream to stimulate a person's immune system to produce antibodies. If the person at some later time is exposed to these viruses or bacteria, the immune system would know immediately which antibodies to produce and would be able to mount a quick counterattack to fight off the disease. Unfortunately, vaccines can also cause the diseases they are meant to protect against. In some people, vaccination can trigger an active infection. These infections are often low-grade and are mistaken for the flu or some other malady and mostly ignored. These organisms can affect the joints.

There are numerous documented cases in both children and adults who have developed acute or chronic arthritis or fibromyalgia immediately after being vaccinated. In fact, as I was gathering research on this topic I was amazed at the number of such reports in the medical literature.[35-51] Only a portion are referenced here. Influenza, measles, mumps, and rubella vaccines seem to be particularly risky in this respect, but that may be because they are so commonly given. Bacillus Calmette-Guérin (BCG) vaccinations, which are used in the treatment of cancer, are also frequently followed by systemic infection and arthritis. Resulting chronic infections may persist for years after the initial vaccination.[52] For patients who already have arthritis or an autoimmune disease, such as lupus, the risk of infection after vaccination is twice as great as that for healthy individuals.[53] The reason for this is that the patient is already infected and the vaccine only adds more infection into the body.

There is an overwhelming amount of evidence to suggest a microbial cause to most forms of arthritis and for fibromyalgia. Whether other factors, such as genetics or hormones, influence the initiation of the disease, it doesn't matter. The fact is, microorganisms are the primary underlying cause.

If arthritis is caused by microorganisms, then you might think the solution would be simple—antibiotics! This approach is usually effective with acute infectious arthritis, but drugs don't usually work for chronic infectious arthritis. If the infection is caused by bacteria, then antibiotics may be helpful. However, if the infection is caused by viruses, fungi, or drug-resistant bacteria, then antibiotics are useless. Even if the problem is caused by antibiotic-sensitive bacteria, drugs may not work. A systemic infection can deposit microbes in areas of the body that are not easily reached by antibiotics or the immune system, allowing them to exist indefinitely. As with Lyme disease, herpes, chicken pox, hepatitis B, candida, and a myriad of other infectious organisms, a chronic remnant of the infection can hold on even after the acute infection is long over. The joints are a favorite gathering spot because of a lack of blood circulation in this area.

Why Haven't Doctors Made the Connection?

If infectious microorganisms are the primary cause for most cases of arthritis, why haven't doctors discovered this? The truth is—they have! Infections have been documented with all the major types of arthritis for many years. The problem is that it is not always easy to identify an active infection with every case of arthritis. This doesn't mean that infections are not present; it means that doctors have not yet been able to conclusively determine the presence of infection in all cases. Doctors tend to be conservative and until there is absolute proof beyond doubt that most all cases of arthritis are caused by infection, they will refrain from making any definitive statement to that effect.

Why is it so hard to identify an infection? Active or acute infections are those cases where the infection has gotten out of hand. The immune system is overwhelmed, and signs of infection are clearly evident. Systemic symptoms such as fever, chills, and nausea often accompany acute infections. The bacterial count in the body and in the infected joints is so high that it is relatively easy to diagnose. However, chronic, localized, low-grade infections are a different matter.

We can have infectious microorganisms living in us without our knowledge and without showing systemic symptoms. The chicken pox virus (varicella-zoster), for example, will cause an acute systemic infection for a few weeks and then go away. The chicken pox virus, however, is never really vanquished from the body; a remnant hides within nerve tissues where it is usually kept from spreading by the immune system. However, whenever the immune system is put under excessive stress, it is unable to adequately contain the virus and it spreads beyond the confines of the nerve tissue and causes another systemic disease called *shingles*. Shingles is common in older people when they undergo a great deal of stress or when they struggle with some other illness.

Herpes is another example. Once a person is infected with herpes, the virus stays for life. Oral herpes (herpes simplex virus) makes itself known by the appearance of fever blisters or cold sores on the lips. Most of the time, the virus remains rather quiet, lurking in nerve roots, but in times of stress or low immunity, it flares up and displays itself prominently on the lips.

We have many microorganisms living in and on our bodies, billions in fact, of all types—bacteria, viruses, and fungi. They live on our skin, in our intestinal tract, and in our mouths. Some even find themselves inside the bloodstream, where they don't belong. It's just a fact of life. There are no tests that can accurately diagnose the presence of all microorganisms in our body. There are tests that can show some of the culprits, but the presence and identity of most organisms remains elusive.

Tracking down infectious organisms in the body isn't always an easy task. One way doctors determine if an infection is present is by counting the number of white blood cells in a blood sample. A normal healthy person has a certain amount of white blood cells per unit volume of blood. If the number of white blood cells is elevated, that gives a

Sting That Pain Away

Are you tired of the constant stabbing pain of arthritis? According to Christopher Kim, MD, medical director of the Monmouth Pain Institute in Red Bank, New Jersey, you can put a stop to arthritis pain with bee venom therapy (BVT). Yes, you can sting that arthritis pain away.

Never heard of bee venom therapy? If you've been stung by a bee, you already have firsthand experience with it. People who use bee venom for medicinal purposes, however, don't wait around for random insect attacks. Using a pair of tweezers, they grasp a living, kicking, stinging, honey bee and put it on their skin. As expected, the skin is harpooned with a barbed venomous stinger. For best results, one sting usually isn't enough. For full therapeutic benefit, you need to be stung 5, 10, or maybe even as many as 80 times every few days. Most doctors usually prefer to inject the venom into their patients rather than use live bees, but many patients prefer to do it the old-fashioned way.

Although a bee sting causes pain, itching, redness, and swelling, many people swear by it, or perhaps at it. Several studies have been published in medical journals on bee venom therapy and many doctors have become bee-lievers. One of them is Christopher Kim, MD. He is a former president of the American Apitherapy Society. Apitherapy (*apis* is Latin for "bee") is the use of bee products for therapeutic purposes. These doctors routinely use BVT for treating arthritis, fibromyalgia, tendonitis, MS, and other painful conditions. The belief is that the venom triggers the release of hormones that deaden the pain and inflammation associated with these conditions. In other words, it is thought to act kind of like a natural non-steroidal anti-inflammatory medication.

Bee venom therapy has been around for centuries. It was supposedly started after beekeepers, who were stung many times, noticed their arthritis pains were relieved. Although not a practice in standard medicine, some doctors have embraced it as an alternative therapy. Many people report good results. Some require bee venom therapy almost daily, but others, after receiving

continued on next page

the initial series of injections or stings, remain pain free for months or years. Apparently, more than just the release of pain-relieving hormones is at work here. Hormones would have only a temporary effect, just as drugs do. And like drugs, don't do anything to solve the underlying problem.

For a more realistic answer, take a closer look at what is really happening. What is bee venom? It's a toxin, a poison, designed to kill and cause pain. When this poison is injected into an arthritic joint, what is going to happen? Keep in mind that the joint is infected with living microorganisms that are causing the arthritis. When these organisms encounter this poison, they die. Once they are killed, joint pain goes away. It's that simple. For some people the relief is only temporary because the joint soon becomes reinfected, but for others the infection is gone for a long time, if not for good.

Most of the research on bee venom therapy has come out of Russia, Japan, and Europe. These studies have clearly demonstrated the antibiotic nature of bee venom.[57-62] Bee venom is described as possessing "highly potent antimicrobial activity." Its bacterial killing power is equal to that of many common antibiotics. In fact, compared to several snake venoms, bee venom was a more effective killing agent on the bacteria being tested. The types of bacteria tested include E. coli, mycobacteria, staphylococci, staphylococci, B. pseudomallei, and spirochetes—all common disease-causing organisms (and also known causes of arthritis). Included among the spirochete bacteria is *Borrelia burgdorferi,* the culprit behind Lyme disease. Because many bacteria are becoming immune to antibiotics, researchers are looking for new drugs that can kill these superbugs. Bee venom is viewed as one of the possible candidates. It kills the superbugs just as easily as the ordinary ones.

One major advantage bee venom has over standard antibiotics is that it also inactivates or inhibits viruses, including leukemia viruses, Herpes simplex virus, and HIV.[63-65]

But that's not all. Bee venom also kills protozoa—single celled parasites that cause diseases like malaria, which is caused by an organism called plasmodium.[66-67] Accounts of bee stings curing malaria victims have been told for ages.

In addition to killing or deactivating microorganisms, the venom is believed to activate processes in the body that improve circulation and stimulate the release of pain-relieving, anti-inflammatory hormones.

In animal studies, bee venom has been proven to be useful as an effective antibiotic and antimicrobial agent.[68] In one study, for instance, young piglets infected with bacterial diarrhea were divided into two groups. One group was treated with standard antibiotic and antidiarrheal drugs for three days. The other group received one bee sting every day for three days. At the end of three days, 90.9 percent of the drug-treated group recovered, and 93.6 percent of the bee-venom group recovered.[69] The bee venom performed better than the drugs.

Bee stings have long been known to ease the pain of rheumatoid arthritis, osteoarthritis, and gout. Since the venom is a potent antibiotic, that makes sense. A number of studies have shown bee venom to be useful in the treatment of various forms of arthritis.[70-74]

In a study with rheumatoid arthritis patients, the results showed a 90 percent positive response, with remarkable improvement in 20 percent of cases, good improvement in 50 percent of cases, and effective improvement in 20 percent of cases. Only 10 percent showed no improvement.[75]

In a study with 70 osteoarthritis patients, the results were similar: 11 cases (15.7 percent) showed excellent improvement; 31 cases (44.3 percent) showed good improvement; 16 cases (22.9 percent) showed some improvement. Only 12 cases (17.1 percent) showed no improvement.[76]

You may not want to rush right out to your nearest bee farm just yet. Some people are highly allergic to bee venom and for them BVT is not an option. For those who are not allergic, treatment can require an initial round of stinging sessions every few days that lasts for several weeks. Thereafter, regular follow-up sessions may be required to keep symptoms under control. Although bee venom therapy may be helpful for some people, it is not the complete answer, as you will learn in the following chapters. ■

clue that an infection might be present. But white blood cell count isn't definitive enough. Sometimes white blood cell levels are high even though there is no active infection. Also, a chronic, low-grade infection can be present without eliciting an unusually high white blood cell response.

Another test is to identify certain antibodies in blood samples. When an infectious organism invades the bloodstream, one of the defensive actions of the immune system is to make antibodies to fight it off. Antibodies are substances that are created to kill one specific type of organism. If you develop the mumps, for example, your body will create antibodies to fight the mumps virus. These antibodies only kill the mumps virus; they have no action against any other type of organism. Therefore, by identifying the types of antibodies present in the blood, doctors know what microorganism is causing the infection. The problem we have with this method is that once a person has been infected and antibodies have been made, the white blood cells keep a memory of the incident and continually produce a small amount of antibodies. So the presence of antibodies in the blood doesn't necessarily indicate an active infection; it only means that at one time in the past the body has encountered this particular organism. You may have had an infection 20 years ago, but you will still have antibodies to that infection running around your bloodstream.

Another problem with relying on antibodies is that there are many organisms that most people encounter at one time in their lives. The presence of antibodies to these organisms is so common that they are expected in the majority of people and, therefore, are overlooked as possible causes. Yet, these common organisms may be the culprits behind the problem. Candida, for example, is a common inhabitant of the human body. Most of us will have antibodies to this fungus, so on analysis, it would be overlooked. Candida, however, is known to cause arthritis.[54-55]

The most diagnostic method for determining the presence of microorganisms is to grow a culture using a sample of blood or synovial fluid. The sample is spread on an agar plate, and whatever is in the fluid is allowed to grow. Whatever grows is then analyzed and identified. One of the problems with this method is that if the microbes are small in number, as would be the case in a chronic arthritic condition, there may be no growth at all. Or, if another common organism is present, it

38

may overpower the real protagonist and prevent it from being identified. Some organisms just don't grow well in cultures and so don't show up, even if they are abundant. These are called noncultivable or uncultivable bacteria. Many of the bacteria that are associated with chronic arthritis are of this type.[56] Another problem is that the growth of organisms varies with temperature, pH, oxygen levels, etc. The culture must be given the right conditions to grow. An anaerobic organism will not grow in an aerobic environment, and likewise an aerobic organism will not grow in an anaerobic environment. Most cultures test for aerobic organisms. However, many arthritic infections are caused by anaerobic organisms. So negative culture results do not necessarily mean microorganisms are not present.

Laboratory tests for infection are not always conclusive. In a study that reviewed 168 confirmed cases of acute infectious arthritis, investigators found that increased white blood cell count occurred in only 40 percent of the cases. Blood cultures failed to show infection 50 percent of the time, while cultures made from synovial fluid missed 12 percent of the time.[78] Therefore, missing the causative agent is not unusual at all. It is even higher with chronic infectious arthritis when the organisms may be present in comparatively small numbers.

The reason why infectious agents have not been found with every case of arthritis is because the methods used to identify the organisms have not been accurate enough. The fact that microorganisms have been found with all the major forms of arthritis, and the fact that infection of the joints is clearly documented as causing arthritis, provide strong evidence for the infection hypothesis.

Another reason why bacteria are not always found in the blood or synovial fluid is because bacteria don't need to be present in these tissues to cause irritation and pain. A chronic, low-grade infection localized in another area of the body may be the source of the problem. This infection may not produce any significant markers for detection, yet can release small quantities of toxic waste material that can have a significant impact on the health of the joints and other tissues. One of the most common sources of chronic infection is the mouth. In the following chapter, you will learn how the health of your mouth is directly related to your joints. This knowledge provides us with the primary cause of arthritis and directs us to the solution.

Chapter 4

The Tooth Connection

A Biting Problem

While medical science has identified several different forms of arthritis, they all have one thing in common. They are all caused or at least exacerbated by microorganisms—bacteria, viruses, and fungi. Where do these microorganisms come from? They can come from just about anywhere. Surprisingly, most joint infections have their origins in the mouth. Microorganisms from oral infections (dental cavities, gum disease, abscesses, etc.) enter the bloodstream, where they take up residence in joint tissues. Here they cause inflammation, swelling, and tissue breakdown, leading to the symptoms characteristic of arthritis.

Our bodies are the home to some 100 trillion bacteria and other microorganisms. Most of them reside in the gastrointestinal tract, but about 10 billion call the mouth their home. There are over 600 species of bacteria that are known to inhabit the human mouth. In addition to all this bacteria, we also have millions of viruses, fungi, and protozoa that thrive alongside them. Although we can't see them with the naked eye, the mouth is teeming with microscopic life.

Some of these organisms live in our mouths without causing too much trouble; others are little hellions, eating away at the teeth, bone, and gums. If they get into the bloodstream, they are capable of spreading their path of destruction throughout the body. Even the more benign organisms that do little harm in the mouth can become devils if they get into the bloodstream. They will do fine in the mouth, causing no harm, but outside their ordinary environment, they can transform from a docile Dr. Jekyll into a destructive Mr. Hyde.

The more destructive organisms in the mouth rot the teeth, infect soft tissues, burrow down into the gums and into the bone, cause inflammation and swelling, create offensive odors, and make the mouth an overall unpleasant nest of infestation. Infection damages tissues allowing microbes to enter capillaries and blood vessels. From here, they circulate though the bloodstream, finding their way into joints and other tissues. If the immune system is strong, most of these invaders are cleaned up without much trouble. If the immune system is compromised in any way or if the source of the infection is pumping large quantities of microbes into the bloodstream, secondary infections can arise in the joints or anywhere in the body.

Oral Health and Arthritis

The connection between oral health and arthritis is not new. It has been recognized since ancient times. References to the coexistence of systemic diseases and toothache are found in ancient Greek and Babylonian medical texts. The Greek physician Hippocrates (460-377 BC), who is known as the father of western medicine, reported curing arthritis by pulling infected teeth.

One of the signers of the Declaration of Independence, Benjamin Rush, MD (1745-1813), was keenly aware of the connection between arthritis and dental health. Dr. Rush served as the Surgeon General of the Continental Army and later as a professor of medicine at the University of Pennsylvania. In his book *Medical Inquiries and Observations* he devoted a chapter to the connection between oral health and systemic disease. In his book he describes a case of rheumatoid arthritis, "Some time in the month of October, 1801," he writes, "I attended Miss A.C. with rheumatism in her hip joint, which yielded, for awhile, to the several remedies for that disease. In the month of November it returned with great violence, accompanied with a severe toothache. Suspecting the rheumatic affection was excited by the pain in her tooth, which was decayed, I directed it to be

41

extracted. The rheumatism immediately left her hip, and she recovered in a few days. She has continued ever since to be free from it."

The connection between oral health and systemic disease was noted by other physicians before him. He states, "I have been made happy by discovering that I have only added to the observations of other physicians, in pointing out a connection between the extraction of decayed and diseased teeth and the cure of general diseases...I cannot help thinking that our success in the treatment of all chronic diseases would be very much promoted, by directing our inquiries into the state of the teeth in sick people."

Doctors and dentists of the nineteenth century frequently observed the coexistence of arthritis with "bad teeth." Extracting infected teeth often led to recovery. This observation led to the proposal of the *focal theory of infection*, which states that an infection in the mouth (or anywhere else in the body) can spread or metastasize and cause secondary infections elsewhere. The primary infection was the focus or the root source of the other infections. Secondary infections could arise anywhere. If the infection affected the heart it could cause endocarditis, a potentially fatal condition; if in the joints it would cause arthritis; likewise, in the gallbladder cholecystitis, the kidneys nephritis, the colon colitis, and so forth.

During the early part of the twentieth century, some of the most distinguished men of medical science published studies on focal infections and their relationship to systemic disease. These early pioneers observed a strong association between dental health and rheumatic diseases. Rheumatic diseases refer to connective tissue disorders and include rheumatoid arthritis, osteoarthritis, rheumatic fever, rheumatic heart disease, psoriatic arthritis, ankylosing spondylitis, fibromyalgia, and systemic lupus erythematosus, among others. Of these, the various forms of arthritis seem to be among the most prominent conditions associated with oral health.

Sir William Willcox, MD (1870-1941), President of the Medical Society of London and Senior Scientific Analyst to the British Home Office, expressed the opinion that 90 percent of non-specific infective arthritis cases were due to infection arising from the teeth.[1]

Russell L. Cecil, MD (1881-1965), who was a professor of clinical medicine at Cornell University Medical School, served as consulting medical director for the Arthritis Foundation, and is considered one of the "Founding Fathers" of American rheumatology stated, "When we come to a consideration of streptococcal infections about the teeth and their relation to systemic disease, we think first and foremost of infectious arthritis and justly so, for so many cases of arthritis in middle and later life are due to dental infection. In our studies on arthritis at Bellevue Hospital, we have frequently succeeded in isolating streptococci from both the blood and joint fluid in patients with infectious arthritis. In some of these patients a streptococcus has also been recovered from the apex (root) of an infected tooth."[2]

One of the most prolific researchers on focal infections was Frank Billings, MD (1854-1932). Dr. Billings was one of the most respected physicians of his time. He was the head of the Department of Medicine of the University of Chicago and served as the President of the American Medical Association. He showed that infections in teeth, gums, and even tonsils can spread throughout the body to ignite arthritis and other health problems. He performed many animal and clinical studies demonstrating the relationship between oral infections and arthritis. Oral infections from the mouth of arthritis patients were injected into animals, which subsequently developed the same form of arthritis. He reported numerous case studies like the following.

Mrs. A.P.R., aged 38, had osteoarthritis of the left hip, which had existed for six years with slight shortening of the leg, pain, stiffness, and lameness on exertion which gradually increased in severity. X-rays showed hip erosion of the head and neck of the femur (upper leg bone) with some flattening of the head. Examination of the woman's mouth revealed a low-grade infection in her tonsils. The tonsils were surgically removed. A culture was grown from the infected tissue. A portion of the culture was then intravenously injected into a laboratory rabbit. Within days the rabbit developed acute multiple osteoarthritis— the same condition the woman suffered from. The infection became so severe that the rabbit died a few days later. Six months after leaving the hospital, Mrs. A.P.R. was free of her arthritis. She could walk, play golf, ride horseback, and perform any physical effort without discomfort. The only vestige of the arthritis was a slight limp due to the shortening of her leg.[3]

43

Another prolific researcher was Weston A. Price, DDS (1870-1948), who served as the Research Director for the American Dental Association. Dr. Price spent 25 years researching the relationship between focal infections in the mouth and systemic disease. In 1923, his research was gathered together and published in a two volume set containing over 1,100 pages.[4] Some of the most thoroughly documented studies in these volumes involved the link between arthritis and oral infections.

One of the cases described by Dr. Price was that of a woman who had such severe deforming arthritis that she had been bedridden for six years and had to be carried into his office. Arthritis affected her knees, hips, spine, neck, and hands. Her hands were so deformed and swollen that she had not been able to feed herself for five years. Several infected teeth were extracted. The patient began to improve immediately. Within three months she was walking with the aid of crutches. In time, she made a complete recovery and no longer needed the crutches. Her hands, which had been "as stiff as castings," limbered up so she could thread needles and sew, an activity she hadn't been able to do for years.

The patient's recovery in itself was remarkable enough, but that wasn't the end of the story. Dr. Price took the infected tooth, washed it thoroughly, and then surgically implanted it underneath the skin of a rabbit. Within two days, the rabbit developed the same type of crippling arthritis as the patient had. After 10 days, it died from the infection.

In another case, a 47-year-old man had received a root canal treatment 23 years prior to seeing Dr. Price. For 14 years he had been suffering from pain and stiffness due to arthritis in his spine, which was progressively growing worse. He was barely able to rotate his body or bend his back from his hips to his head and had been compelled to quit his job. His root canalled tooth had been painful at recurring periods soon after it was filled but had presented no symptoms of discomfort for many years. Suspecting the tooth to be infected, Dr. Price extracted it. The patient made a quick recovery and within six months time felt complete relief from his symptoms and was able to return to work. Nothing was done except removal of the dental infection. Several rabbits inoculated with a culture made from the patient's infected tooth all developed the same deformity of the spine.

44

Dr. Price performed similar studies with thousands of infected teeth from over a thousand patients who were suffering from arthritis and other degenerative diseases. Infected teeth extracted from patients were inserted under the skins of rabbits, and almost invariably, the rabbits immediately developed the same debilitating diseases that the patients had. If a patient came in with arthritis, the rabbits developed arthritis. If the patients had heart conditions or kidney problems, the rabbits developed the same problems, and often others as well. The infections became so severe that the animals usually died within a week or two. In some cases, the infections became so severe that the animals died within 24 hours.

Teeth that caused fatal infections in rabbits were removed, washed, and inserted into other rabbits. These rabbits also died within days from infection. The process was repeated. No matter how many times these teeth were transplanted, the results were similar.

To make sure that the cause of the ill health was due to microbes in the infected teeth, rather than to some other unknown factors, Dr. Price also experimented with inserting sterile teeth under the skin of rabbits. Nothing happened. The rabbits showed no adverse reaction and lived for months without any sign of infection. He even tried inserting objects like coins and still observed no reaction. The rabbits only developed infection when infected teeth or the cultures grown from infected teeth were inserted in the animals.

Dentists often treat the teeth as if they are isolated or disconnected from the rest of the body. Teeth are just as much a part of the body as your heart, lungs, or stomach. If your heart isn't working properly, it can have a pronounced effect on your health. Just like these other organs, anything that affects the teeth can have an effect on the entire body. So, it is not so incredible to believe that if the teeth are sick, the rest of the body will feel the effects.

One of the effects of oral infection is a change in blood chemistry. Calcium levels, red and white blood cell counts, pH balance, blood sugar, coagulation time, and a whole host of antibodies and inflammation markers are influenced by oral infections. The blood becomes more acidic, blood sugar (glucose) increases, red blood cells decline—all of these changes can have adverse effects on health. Another substance that is influenced by oral infection is uric acid. Normal uric acid levels are disrupted by dental infections. A study of cases before and after the removal of dental infection has shown a reduction of uric acid following the removal of dental infections.[5] Elevated blood uric acid promotes the development of sodium urate crystals in the joints. Urate crystals are the characteristic feature of gout. This provides further evidence that infection is the underlying cause of gout.

Although bacteria themselves may attack tissues and cause many changes in the blood, a bigger problem is the toxins they produce. The bacteria don't even need to be in the bloodstream to cause trouble. Infection in a tooth can release a continual stream of toxins that drain into the blood, slowly poisoning the body. Certain tissues, such as the joints, may be highly sensitive to some of these toxins and will be the first to react or become irritated. Therefore, joint and muscle pain can arise even though there are no actual bacteria in these tissues.

Modern Science and the Tooth Connection

The link between oral health and arthritis has been documented for many years. Research on focal infections continues to this day. On Medline, a computer database of medical journal articles, there are over 400 studies published since 1980 with the search parameters of "arthritis and periodontal disease." Let's take a look at some of the recent research findings.

The bacterium *Porphyromonas gingivalis* (P. gingivalis), as the name implies, is one of the most common causes of gingivitis and periodontitis (i.e., gum disease). It is a normal inhabitant of the mouth. Virtually everyone has P. gingivalis living in their mouths to some extent. Of course, those people who have active gum infections have an overgrowth of this organism. And the more you have in your mouth, the more likely it is that it will find its way into your bloodstream and end up in other parts of the body, such as your joints.

Antibodies to P. gingivalis are more commonly found in those with rheumatoid arthritis than among the general population. In fact, an oral infection from P. gingivalis is a recognized risk factor for rheumatoid arthritis.[6]

P. gingivalis isn't the only troublemaker. Any number of thousands of species of bacteria, viruses, and fungi that inhabit the mouth can potentially infect the joints. A number of oral bacteria have been found

46

in the blood and in the synovial fluid of patients afflicted with rheumatoid and other forms of arthritis. The presence of oral bacteria in the blood and joint fluids indicates that the bacteria migrate from the mouth, through the bloodstream, and into the joints, where they are trapped and initiate the series of events that leads to the symptoms characteristic of various forms of arthritis.[7] The medical literature is filled with cases where oral bacteria have caused arthritis.[8-10]

Studies show that people with gum disease are eight times more likely than the general population to have rheumatoid arthritis.[11] Conversely, people with arthritis are more likely to have gum disease and missing teeth.[12-13]

Numerous studies have confirmed a close relationship between periodontal disease and rheumatoid and juvenile arthritis.[14-19] Evidence also shows a strong relationship between the severity of periodontal disease and rheumatoid arthritis. Those people with advanced rheumatoid arthritis are more likely to experience more significant periodontal problems compared to the general population.[20]

The disease processes in both arthritis and gum disease are very similar. "Both rheumatoid arthritis and periodontal disease," says rheumatologist Elliot Rosenstein, MD, a professor of medicine at New York University, "are characterized by self-sustaining inflammation in a fluid-filled compartment adjacent to bone, in which inflammatory cells and other factors lead to common clinical manifestations (pain, swelling, tenderness) and, eventually, to erosion of the adjacent bone."[21] In essence, the disease process in both cases is the same.

The relationship between arthritis and periodontal disease is more than just a shared susceptibility. For example, when arthritis is induced in lab animals, they often develop periodontal disease as well.[22] The similarities don't stop there. Oral bacteria that cause gum disease produce the same autoimmune markers in the blood that characterize rheumatoid arthritis.[23-24]

The similarities between rheumatoid arthritis and gum disease are so strong that some researchers claim that they are both expressions of the same disease.[25] Although this may sound strange at first, it really makes a lot of sense. The tooth and socket comprise a joint, just as the vertebrae or elbow form joints. Whether you have arthritis in your finger or knee joints or in the joints of your teeth, it is all the same.

Normal Joint

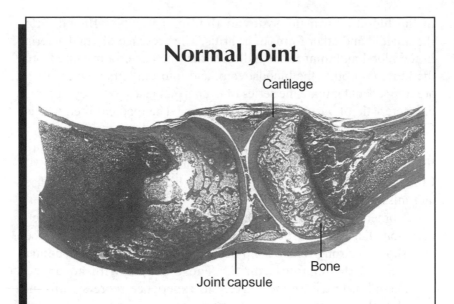

Cartilage

Joint capsule

Bone

Photographs show the articulating surfaces of a normal and an arthritic knee joint of a rabbit. The photo on the right was taken at a slightly different plane from the photo on the left and shows part of the ligament connecting the upper and lower leg bones.

An infected human tooth, which had been root canalled, was extracted from the patient. A culture was grown from bacteria inside the tooth. This culture was injected into the rabbit. Within 12 days the animal developed swelling in its left knee and began to have difficulty moving that leg. After 24 days the animal was put down and autopsied.

The photo on left shows the rabbit's right knee joint, which was unaffected by the infection and appears to be normal. Note the good condition of the joint tissues. The heads of the leg bones and cartilage covering them have smooth, even surfaces and the synovial membranes and joint capsule are intact and clearly defined.

The photo on right shows the rabbit's arthritic left knee joint. Note the extensive degeneration caused by the infection.

Arthritic Joint

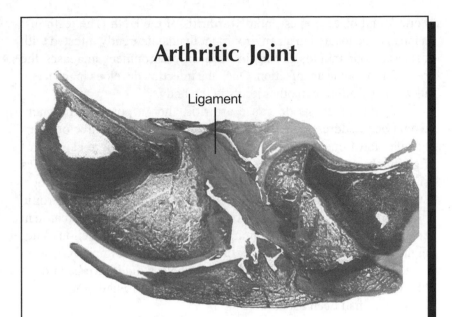

Ligament

A difference in size between the two joints is due to swelling in the affected knee. In the arthritic joint there has been very extensive inflammatory destruction of the joint capsule, with its rupture. The pus escaped when the tissues were prepared. The internal structure of the head of the leg bone shows decalcification and the articulating surfaces and their cartilages have been very seriously mutilated by the inflammatory process. The attachments of the connecting ligament have been seriously injured and its body is undergoing necrosis.

This damage was caused in just 24 days from bacteria removed from an extracted human tooth. The amount of bacteria that was inoculated into the rabbit was miniscule, weighing no more than one or two thousandths of a gram. Despite the body's natural defenses against infection, the bacteria were able to survive in the bloodstream and invade the joint tissue. Bacteria entering the bloodstream from infected teeth in the mouth can have a similar effect.

Periodontal disease is essentially arthritis of the teeth. The teeth just happen to be located in an environment that is inherently infested with bacteria—our mouths. Being in such an environment increases the risk of developing an infection. Once the infection develops in the teeth, it can easily migrate to other joints in the body.

If oral infections do cause arthritis, then a possible treatment would be to address dental issues. If you remove the source or focus of infection from the mouth, then the body will be more capable of fighting the remaining infection in the rest of the body. Recent studies show that this is exactly what happens. In one such study, for instance, subjects with rheumatoid arthritis and mild-to-moderate chronic periodontitis of at least three years' duration received dental treatment consisting of scaling/root planning and oral hygiene instruction. After eight weeks, 59 percent of the patients demonstrated improvement in standard arthritis tests.[26] The results probably would have been even higher if all dental issues were addressed and additional oral hygiene techniques had been used.

In regards to fibromyalgia, infection is likely the underlying cause. However, instead of attacking the joints, the microorganisms attack primarily the nerves and central nervous system. Various microorganisms have been linked to fibromyalgia, including oral bacteria.[27]

Numerous studies, both recent and past, have provided convincing evidence that treating dental issues can have a pronounced effect on systemic health. Drugs used to treat arthritis and fibromyalgia don't do a thing to stop the progression of the disease; they only mask the symptoms. Addressing dental issues, on the other hand, actually causes a regression of the disease and offers the possibility of a complete recovery.

Joint Replacement

With standard drug therapy, symptoms may abate, but the disease continues to progress. As the disease worsens, at some point joint replacement is usually offered. Joint replacement is depicted as a wonderful solution to all joint problems. No more pain, more freedom of movement, and on and on; it all sounds very enticing.

Besides the fact that artificial joints are only temporary and may need to be replaced in a few years, there is another very important limitation—they are also highly prone to infection. Joints are already highly susceptible to infection, but when natural tissue is cut out and replaced with artificial structures, the degree of susceptibility skyrockets. You have just traded an infection in a natural joint for an infection in an artificial one. The problem with the artificial joint is that plastic and metal can't fight off infection or heal themselves like living tissue can.

Artificial joints are commonly infected by oral bacteria—further evidence that oral bacteria tend to migrate to joint tissues. Dental procedures often cause gums to bleed. Bleeding gums are wounds, just like any other wound you would get on your skin. They provide a portal for infectious organisms to enter into your bloodstream. Even if the wound heals within a couple of days, this is long enough to allow bacteria to enter and attack the joints, causing acute infection. Those people who have artificial joints are especially susceptible to infection after having dental work.[28]

Orthopedic surgeons routinely recommend that patients with artificial joints receive antibiotics when they have *any* dental work done, even routine cleaning.[29-30] Antibiotics should be given before the dental work is performed and then again afterward. Even with the administration of antibiotics, there is no guarantee that an infection won't occur. Not everyone who visits the dentist needs antibiotics. If you are free of arthritis, don't have artificial joints or other devices (e.g., mechanical heart valves, artificial eye, etc.), and your health is not otherwise compromised, then your immune system should be capable of withstanding the amount of bacteria that seeps into your bloodstream after dental work.

It is interesting that any prosthetic device implanted inside the body has an increased potential for infection. This would also include dental implants, crowns, and root canalled teeth. In these cases, they are right in the center of a source of bacteria and, therefore, are prime targets for infection. They can themselves become the foci for infection.

Chapter 5

The Root of the Problem

The Anatomy of a Tooth

The adult human mouth has 32 teeth—12 molars (including four wisdom teeth), eight premolars (also called *bicuspids*), four canines, and eight incisors. The incisors are the front teeth and are used for cutting food. The molars' primary function is to masticate food. Molars have two to four roots while the other teeth have a single root. The roots fit into a hole or socket in the jawbone. The teeth are held in place by the periodontal membrane and the gums.

The part of the tooth that projects above the gum line is called the *crown*. It is covered in a thick, hard material called *enamel*. Enamel needs to be hard and durable to withstand the pressure of chewing and to resist chemical and biological action that might otherwise harm the tooth.

Below the gum line and surrounding the root of the tooth, the enamel becomes very thin. This part of the enamel is called *cementum*. Cementum is connected to the periodontal membrane that helps hold the tooth in the socket.

Beneath the layer of enamel is the *dentin*, which makes up the majority of the structure of the tooth. Chemically it is very similar to bone.

At the center of the tooth is a cavity containing the nerves and blood vessels that feed the tooth. This is called the *pulp*.

Our teeth are located in an environment that can be hostile. They are surrounded by a multitude of disease-causing bacteria, bathed in acids, and subjected to crushing forces. Despite all this, the teeth are very durable and are designed to last a lifetime, and they will, if they are cared for properly. However, for various reasons, teeth may succumb to negative influences and develop infection. Infection may be in the teeth themselves (these are commonly called dental cavities) or they may be in the surrounding soft tissue (gum or periodontal disease).

The Human Tooth

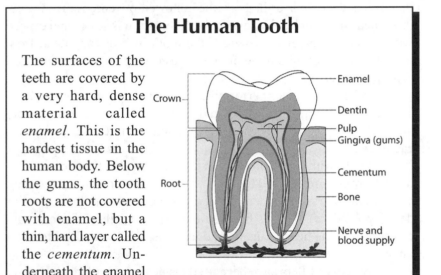

The surfaces of the teeth are covered by a very hard, dense material called *enamel*. This is the hardest tissue in the human body. Below the gums, the tooth roots are not covered with enamel, but a thin, hard layer called the *cementum*. Underneath the enamel and cementum lies the *dentin*. Dentin is less hard than enamel and cementum, and similar in composition to bone. It makes up the majority of the tooth. At the center of the tooth is the *pulp*, which contains the nerve and blood vessels.

Root Canals

Small cavities are usually treated by cleaning out the infection and filling the void with a hard material. If the infection penetrates deep into the tooth and affects the pulp, a simple patch will not work.

Once bacteria reach the pulp the integrity of the tooth is lost. Blood provides a rich source of nourishment for bacteria, so the infection rapidly multiplies within the pulp chamber. From here it is easy for the infection to enter the bloodstream and spread. Infection in the pulp is invariably fatal to the tooth.

The dentist has the option of either pulling the diseased tooth or performing a root canal. At this point, the tooth is too far gone to be saved alive. The root canal procedure creates a dummy tooth using the shell of the original. No artificial tooth could fill the void as precisely as the tooth that naturally occupies that position. So, the tooth remains in position, the pulp is drilled out, the hollowed-out core is disinfected, then filled with a rubber-like material, and finally, it is sealed and capped with a gold or porcelain crown. If the tooth isn't already dead from the infection, drilling out the pulp and destroying its nerve and blood supply seals its fate.

Dentists have been performing root canals for over 150 years. They are among the most common dental procedures. Approximately 40 million root canal procedures are performed in the United States each year.

Patients with heart problems such as valvular heart disease or heart murmurs are advised to take antibiotics as a preventive measure against infection when undergoing a root canal treatment (or any major dental procedure). This is because bacteria from the infected tooth can spread to the heart, causing endocarditis, which can lead to heart failure.

A variety of fillers have been used inside root canalled teeth. Over the years, one of the challenges facing dentists has been finding a suitable filler, one that does not expand or contract as it hardens. Contraction would leave empty space inside the root canal, and expansion could crack the tooth. Originally, root canals were filled with gold or amalgam (an alloy of mercury, tin, silver, and copper). The most common filler today is gutta percha, a resin from the isonandra gutta tree, which comes from the Malay Peninsula. Some fillers, such as Sargenti paste (also known as N2), contain paraformaldehyde (a powder form of formaldehyde) and sometimes mercury or lead. The purpose of these poisons is to continue the process of disinfecting the tooth even after the dental work is complete. Unfortunately, these toxins can seep out of the root tip and into the bloodstream, causing damage to the bones, liver, and brain.

In theory, a root canalled tooth, with a suitable filling material, should perform the function of masticating foods about as well as a living tooth. Tooth decay is arrested, the tooth is "saved" and the patient maintains a bright, healthy smile. However, looks can be deceiving.

The Problem with Sterilization

Before receiving a root canal treatment, the diseased tooth may be very painful. After the procedure, the pain goes away and the tooth is considered "saved." However, root canals are deceptive. The absence of pain is not an indication of health. Root canalled teeth no longer hurt because the nerve has been removed. The tooth is now dead. Dead tissues don't feel pain.

During root canal treatment, the infected cavity of the tooth is thoroughly washed and disinfected to remove and kill all microbes. When filling material is put into the cavity, it is assumed that the tooth is now sterilized. Therefore, infection should no longer be a problem. Right? Unfortunately, this is not the case. No matter how much care is taken to remove microorganisms, a root canalled tooth will *always* remain infected.

The very nature of the tooth does not allow complete sterilization while it still resides in the mouth. Let me explain why. Most people tend to think of teeth as solid chunks of calcium, like a rock. Teeth, however, are not as solid as they appear but are very porous. Even the hard enamel coating is filled with pores.

Dentin, which makes up the bulk of the tooth, is filled with millions of tiny, hollow tubes called *tubules*. If you took one small front tooth and could place all the tubules end to end, they would extend for three miles. That's how much space you have in each of your teeth (see photo on following page).

Bacteria are small enough that they can easily enter and take up residence within the tubules. Sugar and electrolytes are also small enough to fit into the tubules, so the bacteria have access to plenty of nutrients to feed on. The long, narrow channels constituting the dental tubules, with their multiple branches produce a structure particularly

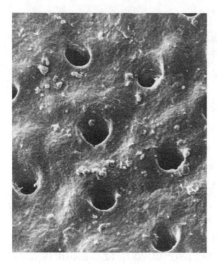

The dentin in teeth are filled with tubular pores called tubules.

favorable for the hiding away of these organisms because of the mechanical difficulty of getting disinfectants into the structure.

This problem was brought to light during the focal infection research of Weston A. Price. He discovered that even though root canalled teeth may show no obvious signs of infection while in the patient's mouth, when the teeth are extracted, washed, and inserted under the skin of rabbits, the animals develop severe infections. Since his studies showed that sterile teeth cause no infection, he began to suspect that many, if not all, root canalled teeth may be infected. This prompted him to design a series of experiments to demonstrate why this may be so.

One of his earliest tests was to place in the roots of canalled and disinfected teeth a sterile root dressing that was soaked in various antiseptics. The teeth containing the dressing and antiseptics were then sealed, just as they would be in a normal root canal procedure. The soaking of the root dressing with antiseptic chemicals insured that the root canal was thoroughly sterilized and would remain so for a period of time after the procedure. This first series of tests was done on human volunteers.

Anywhere from 24 to 48 hours after the procedure, the dressings were removed from the teeth. Many different types of disinfecting

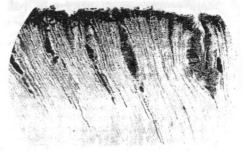

Left. Cross section of a portion of dentin. Bacteria, identified by the dark streaks, are seen here growing inside dental tubules.

Right. Bacteria penetrate deep into the dentin along the tubules of the tooth and work their way toward the tooth's pulp. Notice the extensive decay at the top of this cross secton.

chemicals were used to see which were most effective. When the dressings were examined, Dr. Price states, "To our amazement, in practically all dressings that were left in roots 48 hours, and with most of them after 24 hours, the dressing was found infected regardless of what disinfectant was used on the dressing." The antiseptics used in the dressings very rapidly lost their disinfecting power and after only a day to two were teeming with infection.

In another series of experiments, Price took already extracted teeth that were infected and performed root canal treatments on them, drilling out the pulp and disinfecting them as is normally done. He then implanted the "sterilized" teeth under the skin of rabbits. The animals all died from the resulting infections.

57

Price tested the germ-killing ability of over 100 different antiseptic substances, including hydrogen peroxide, iodine, formaldehyde, and sulfuric acid. None of them were completely satisfactory in disinfecting teeth, even when the amount used was so large that if used on patients it would cause serious injury.

Price states, "We have tested a number of disinfectants by treating the teeth with them before planting them under the skin of a rabbit, as nearly as possible as they would be treated in the mouth. In this way we have tested many disinfectants. I have now made several hundred of these determinations, results of which emphasize the need both for a new appreciation of the danger from infected teeth, because of the apparent difficulty, if not impossibly, for sterilizing infected teeth by treating through a root canal."

Price found that one of the most effective disinfectants was formalin (containing 40 percent formaldehyde). He soaked an infected tooth in formalin for 15 minutes, more than enough time to kill any infection on the surface or in the cavity of the tooth. He then thoroughly washed the tooth to remove all traces of the chemical and inserted it under the skin of a rabbit. The tooth still caused infection. He concluded, "It is exceedingly difficult to neutralize infected dentin under any circumstances without using medicament which may in some degree endanger the supporting structures."

The tubules in the dentin of the teeth form an intricate network of channels and canals. This labyrinth makes it difficult to sterilize a tooth even when it is totally immersed in disinfectants. Price demonstrated that no disinfectant is capable of penetrating deep enough into the tubules to completely sterilize the teeth. The only way he could assure teeth were completely sterilized was to boil them in water. Boiled teeth did not cause infection in the lab animals.

Dr. Price extracted hundreds of root canalled teeth, and in every case, the teeth were infected. Often the patients complained of pain, tenderness, or swelling, and the infection could be identified on X-rays. But in many cases, there were no signs of infection, no pain, and no evidence on X-rays. Yet, when the teeth were extracted it was clear that they were, indeed, infected.

Although Price's experiments were conducted many years ago, what he discovered is still valid—all root canalled teeth remain infected. Critics argue that root canal techniques have greatly improved

58

over the years, and today, they are safe and effective. Yet, even today, root canalled teeth are often so infected and painful that they need to be pulled. Techniques apparently have not improved all that much. In fact, the disinfectants used are basically the same as those tested by Price and found to be ineffective. Even the major filling material, gutta percha, is the same.

George E. Meining, DDS, who spent much of his career as an endodontist (root canal specialist), states that despite the technical advances in dentistry since Price's time, "The underlying problem still exists; bacteria are live inside the tooth. Antibiotics and disinfectants do not get rid of them. No root canalled tooth is free from potentially harmful bacteria. It is safer to pull a severely diseased tooth rather than plug and cap it, forming a breeding ground of decay, sealing in poisons and bacteria that will leak into the bloodstream for the rest of your life."[1]

A Bacterial Fortress

Our body's most effective weapon against infection is our immune system's army of white blood cells. There are several different types of white blood cells, each of which has a slightly different function. When a white blood cell comes into contact with a foreign body, such as invading bacteria, it releases chemical signals that trigger inflammation and cause other white blood cells to rush toward the invader. These cells can literally eat bacteria, which are then broken down by substances inside the cells. Other white blood cells attack bacteria by releasing substances which are toxic to the foreign organisms. And others produce antibodies custom designed to kill that particular invader.

Despite the immune system's formidable defensive force, the white blood cells are completely baffled and helpless when it comes to the matter of fighting off an infection inside the dentin of a tooth. White blood cells and their products cannot penetrate into the dentin to attack the bacteria.

In the tubules, the bacteria are completely protected from the body's defensive forces. The tooth, in essence, becomes an impenetrable fortress, where the bacteria can live and even thrive without molestation.

At the same time, bacteria expel toxins, waste products that can have very detrimental effects on surrounding tissues and on health in general. This can, but not always, be evidenced by a local infection (usually low grade and chronic) or a systemic involvement, such as arthritis (infection of the joints), endocarditis (infection of the heart), nephritis (infection of the kidneys), or some other condition.

As the bacteria in the tubules grow and crowd each other, some migrate out of their protective lair and find their way into the bloodstream. Here they can travel throughout the body. If not arrested by the patrolling white blood cells, the bacteria can lodge in most any tissue or organ and begin a new colony. Bacteria tend to collect in areas where the blood supply is restricted and the immune response is slow. One of the prime locations is in the joints. Joints don't have a blood supply like other body tissues, providing a good opportunity for settlement. If the joint has experienced trauma involving tissue injury that has not completely healed, bacteria find it a particularly favorable site to infest.

Most of the time, the white blood cells do a good job of tracking down these renegade bacteria and keeping them under control. Systemic effects may be mild or not even present. If the immune system is put under undue stress, however, these invaders can run wild.

What about antibiotics? Can't they be used to fight the infection? Unfortunately, they too are helpless. A root canalled tooth no longer has a blood supply, therefore, neither white blood cells nor antibiotics can get inside.

The dead (i.e., root canalled) tooth, says Dr. Price "furnishes an environment which is particularly favorable to the invading organism and unfavorable to the host, in that the former is protected from the aggressive defensive forces of the latter, while able, by the natural laws governing the behavior of liquids and gases, to secure a continuous supply of nutriment through the walls of the fort."

This fort makes the root canalled tooth a breeding ground—a focus—of infection. For this reason, placing an infected tooth beneath the skin of a rabbit is many times more dangerous to the rabbit than injecting it with the same quantity of pure bacteria. Pure bacteria would be completely vulnerable to attack from the body's defensive forces. However, a root canalled tooth can spread infection with invincibility.

The rabbit (or human) is helpless. In the majority of instances, the rabbits in Price's experiments died within two weeks.

Toxic Shock Syndrome

The most common site for focal infections is in the mouth, but they can occur anywhere in the body. Toxic shock syndrome (TSS) is perhaps the most readily recognized condition associated with focal infections. In his book *The Roots of Disease*, Robert Kulacz, DDS, makes an excellent comparison between root canal treated teeth and, believe it or not, tampons.

Toxic shock syndrome is a potentially fatal illness caused by bacterial toxins that circulate in the bloodstream. It was first identified in the late 1970s and almost exclusively associated with woman who used superabsorbent tampons. While different types of bacteria can cause TSS, the most common are *Staphylococcus aureus* and *Streptococcus pyogenes* (which, by the way, also commonly infect root canalled teeth).

Symptoms include fever, muscle aches, chills, and malaise (a general feeling of discomfort, uneasiness, or ill health). Other symptoms may also include headache, cough, nausea, diarrhea, abdominal pain, confusion or disorientation, and low blood pressure. Toxic shock syndrome can affect any organ in the body, including the lungs, liver, kidneys, heart, and pancreas. Death can result from multiple organ failure.

These superabsorbent tampons can be viewed, in a sense, as if they were large, sterile, root canalled teeth. But, instead of being inserted under the skin of rabbits, they end up in the female reproductive tract and quickly become infected.

Like root canalled teeth, tampons provide an ideal environment for bacterial growth. In its warm, dark, moist position in the reproductive tract, the porous tampon allows bacteria to seep in along with blood that serves as a rich source of nourishment. If the tampon is left in place for too long, the bacteria can multiply in large numbers. Bacteria, and the toxins they produce, find their way into the bloodstream and spread throughout the body. The bacteria can take hold in other parts of the body causing secondary infections.

61

Antibiotics are useless as long as the tampon remains in place. The body's own defense system, likewise, is helpless. There is no blood supply into the tampon where the bacteria are breeding. Therefore, the white blood cells that normally fight disease-causing microorganisms cannot get to the focal point of the infection and neither can antibiotics. The only way to fight the infection is to first remove the source of the infection—the tampon. Once the source is removed, then antibiotics and the immune system have a chance at fighting off the remaining infection and clearing out the toxins.

TSS can also arise from infected teeth, whether they are root canalled or not. For example, a nine-year-old girl, who was not using tampons, developed TSS. Her symptoms included arthralgia (joint pain without inflammation) and myalgia (muscle pain), which progressed to renal failure. The problem was traced to her upper-right canine tooth. The tooth had not been root canalled, but it was badly abscessed.[2]

Root canals aren't the only potential troublemakers. They are prime suspects because of their nature, but any tooth can become infected and act as a focus of infection.

Stress as a Contributing Factor

Do all root canals cause arthritis? Not necessarily. The probability that a root canal will trigger a secondary infection, such as arthritis, depends primarily on two conditions: (1) the quality of the root canal and (2) the health of the patient.

If the root canal was not thoroughly cleaned and disinfected or not properly filled and capped, then the chances that the tooth will become badly infected are great. The more infection a tooth holds, the more likely it is to cause systemic involvement.

Even today, with modern dental techniques and materials, not all root canals are of equal quality. Dentists, like in any profession, vary in their professional skills and precision. Consequently, many root canals are substandard and prone to infection.

If the patient's health is compromised and the immune system is incapable of completely containing the infection in a root canalled tooth, then there is also an increased risk of systemic involvement.

A person who has many health problems or is subjected to excess stress is more likely to experience a secondary reaction from an infected tooth, whether it is root canalled or not. In contrast, a person in good health may experience no systemic problems because his or her immune system is fully capable of dealing with the infection in the tooth. However, multiple dental infections can overwhelm the body, even if it is strong.

There are many factors that can influence health: excessive stress at school or work, divorce, death of a loved one, loss of employment, family troubles, pregnancy, illness, physical exhaustion, exposure to toxins or pollution, chronic dehydration, poor diet, sugar addiction, and the use of tobacco, alcohol, or drugs. All of these conditions can adversely affect your immune system and lower your defense against infection. The onset of arthritis often surfaces after a stressful event in a person's life.

Dr. Price describes the case of a 20-year-old woman who came to him for dental work and received crowns on some of her teeth. She later came down with typhoid fever and immediately afterward developed arthritis. He followed her case for 28 years, and during most of that time, she became progressively worse until she was entirely unable to walk. Becoming suspicious that the crowns she had received years before may be harboring infection and be contributing to her problem, he removed the infected teeth. From that moment on her arthritis progressively got better.

An overload of an infectious nature can lower the body's defenses to such an extent that a previously controlled dental infection will intensify to the point that it can lead to systemic involvement.

Dr. Price witnessed many patients who, after experiencing some great trauma in their lives, soon after developed arthritis or some other health problem. He designed an experiment to verify what he observed in his patients. He injected four rabbits with a culture derived from an infected tooth of a patient who was suffering from arthritis. The amount injected into the rabbits was small enough that, under ordinary circumstances, the animals would have little difficulty fighting off the infection and would remain healthy. Two of the rabbits served as controls and two as the test subjects. For the next 32 days, the two test rabbits were subjected to stress by being exposed to cold temperatures for 15 minutes every day or two. The two control animals were kept in a warm cage without exposure to cold.

The two rabbits that were kept in a warm cage showed no adverse effects from the inoculations of bacteria, even after several months. The two that were exposed to the chilling temperatures, however, developed very severe multiple arthritis. This experiment provided the proof that stress can lower resistance to infection enough to allow even a small amount of bacteria to cause arthritis.

Dr. Price observed that infectious illnesses, particularly influenza, often lowered a person's resistance enough to cause the infection in a bad tooth to affect the entire body. He also witnessed many women develop arthritis after becoming pregnant, which can be an enormously stressful time. He assumed that one of the reasons why women experience arthritis more often than men is because of pregnancy.

Dental infections, while potentially harmful, may not be causing apparent or serious injury until the individual is subjected to some other overload, at which time a serious break may come. The chief contributing overloads are influenza, pregnancy, lactation, malnutrition, exposure, grief, worry, fear, and age.

A person who has an unresolved dental infection carries, as Dr. Price describes, "a potential charge of dynamite," which may, when least expected, explode and affect the health of his or her entire body. If you are young and healthy with few stresses in your life, then properly performed root canals will probably have little effect on you. However, we all age, and no matter how healthy you are, as you age your resistance to infection declines. So the root canal that never troubled you when you were 30 years old may become a curse to you as you approach 70.

Severity of Oral Infection Does Not Equate to the Degree of Systemic Involvement

After learning how oral infections can influence overall health, it would seem logical to assume that the greater the severity of an oral infection, the more influence it will have on health. Therefore, severe oral infections should be accompanied by major health problems or pronounced arthritis. This, however, is not the case.

What might seem like a paradox of the focal infection concept is the observation that people with severely acute oral infections do not necessarily display any other health problems, while people who have minor or no apparent dental problems often do.

You cannot tell simply by looking at the mouth to what degree the body is absorbing toxins and bacteria. Generally, if an acute infection is present, this indicates that the body is strong enough to cause marked symptoms, which are a part of the healing process. It is when the symptoms are mild and chronic that the most harm is done. When a person develops an abscess, the pain can be intense and pus may even drain from a fistula—an opening in the gums. Then gradually, the pain may fade away and the fistula heals over. The absence of pain and pus does not necessarily mean the problem has suddenly disappeared or that the infection has gone away. It can mean that the body is no longer capable of sustaining an adequate defense to expel the toxins in a proper manner. The infection has become chronic, and the pus and toxins are now draining into the bloodstream, where they irritate and break down the person's most susceptible tissues.

Dr. Price describes this situation, "We have very frequently seen, and this can be observed in many mouths, the scar of a fistula which has closed, not because the conditions have become better though they apparently have, since the flow has stopped, but because the conditions have become worse…Since an adequate active defense against a dental infection produces a vigorous local reaction with attending extensive absorption, and the products of inflammatory reaction— namely, exudates and plasma in sufficient quantity to require an overflow, usually spoken of as pus from a fistula—this overflow may be, and usually is, evidence of an active defense and is constituted almost wholly of neutralized products, and is often sterile; and such a condition is much more safe than the same infected tooth without such an active local reaction."

Dr. Price describes a patient with a fistula that would occasionally close; the tooth would become tender; the fistula would open, establishing free discharge into the mouth; and the tenderness would subside. Price insisted the patient have the tooth removed. The patient timidly agreed but always delayed the operation for fear of following through with the procedure. The fistula eventually closed, the tooth ceased to become tender, and the area appeared to heal. With the troubling symptoms gone, the patient saw no immediate need to go back to the dentist and stayed away for a couple of years. It was after the patient began to develop symptoms of arthritis that he began to reconsider. Finally, he consented to the removal of the tooth. The tooth was pulled and found to still be infected. Once the tooth was gone, the patient's arthritis symptoms were soon greatly relieved.

In another case, a middle-aged man with properly performed root canals expressed no signs of pain or discomfort. He could eat without thought or consideration. He, however, suffered from arthritis, and for months walked with great difficulty. The pain became so severe that he was unable to work. With the removal of the root canalled teeth, his symptoms completely vanished. In a follow-up visit five years later, he was still free from pain.

Dentists can spot infection beneath the gums using X-rays. Infection presents itself as a faint halo around the apex of the tooth. The absence of this halo is generally interpreted as indicating that no infection is present. However, many teeth without clear evidence of infection on X-rays have proven to be infected. So X-rays are not foolproof.

Dr. Price found that even very seriously infected teeth may give no physical symptoms (absence of pain or inflammation) or evidence on X-rays. Price describes such a case. A man had rheumatoid arthritis, which crippled him so severely that he could walk only by shuffling his feet. His hands were equally helpless. With the removal of his root canalled teeth, his arthritic symptoms, which he had had for some time, "entirely and quickly disappeared" and did not return.[3]

While abscesses and other acute infections may be severe, the infections that don't cause much or any pain can cause the greatest amount of systemic trouble. These infections are chronic, quiet, and destructive.

Bad Teeth Attract Infection

Dead and diseased teeth are magnets for infection. Microorganisms are attracted to them because once inside the teeth, they can exist indefinitely, receiving a continual source of nourishment

66

while being protected from the body's defenses and against medications. Any type of infectious organism can find safe haven in these teeth.

Diseased teeth can harbor not only harmful *oral* bacteria, but other invaders as well. Any infectious microorganism that gets into the bloodstream can find its way to the mouth and eventually locate those teeth that do not have an adequate defense. Therefore, any systemic infection can leave a vestige of itself in a dead tooth, even after the primary infection is long gone. This may help explain why symptoms from certain infections seem to linger for months or years. Lyme disease, for instance, can cause an acute infection, but once it is gone, symptoms such as arthritis can last indefinitely.

Dr. Price cites a case of a woman who while in the tropics was infected with malaria. Medical treatment cured her of the disease. Over the following years, however, she had periodic relapses of the disease, even though she lived in Ohio, an area free from malaria. She went to Dr. Price for dental work. He removed a bad tooth. Whenever a dentist removes infected teeth or does any major dental work, microorganisms in the mouth are invariably released into the body. Almost immediately, she developed a violent and typical attack of malaria. Her condition was positively diagnosed by the identification of the organism in her blood. The infection was treated, and she recovered as she normally did. Prior to her dental treatment, she had experienced frequent relapses of the disease. After the removal of her infected tooth, the relapses abruptly stopped and never reoccurred.

In another case, a man had three infected teeth removed. Bacteria cultures were made from each tooth and injected into three male rabbits. In this case, the development of arthritis wasn't a surprise, but what was a surprise was that each of the rabbits developed an infection in its testes. On being questioned, the patient's reply was "Can't a person have any secrets?" He confessed that he had been infected with gonorrhea 20 years previously and had been treated and supposedly cured. Even after 20 years, the bacteria still lived inside him, apparently in his teeth.

As mentioned in an earlier chapter, gonorrhea, syphilis, and other venereal diseases are known to cause arthritis. Arthritis usually develops after or during the acute infection and can become chronic.

Urinary tract infections are also responsible for many cases of arthritis.[4] Infectious organisms that cause measles, strep throat, pneumonia, rheumatic fever, meningitis, and gastroenteritis (stomach flu), to mention a few, are known to cause arthritis.

If you have root canalled teeth, virtually any infection you encounter in life can hide undetected inside them, all the while releasing toxins and causing reactions that adversely affect blood chemistry and the immune system.

The Solution
Remove the Underlying Problem

The cause of arthritis is known. So what's the solution? The first step is to identify and eliminate any focus of infection—the root of the problem. This infection could be in the bowels, urinary tract, sex organs, mouth, and really almost anywhere. In the vast majority of cases, however, the focus is in the mouth, specifically in and around the teeth.

Using antibiotics to kill bacteria in the joints and teeth would be a logical approach but doesn't always work. Infections in dead and severely diseased teeth don't respond well to antibiotics.

When a doctor treats a patient with severely diseased or dead tissue, what course is usually taken? The only solution is amputation. Just like a gangrenous limb, dead and diseased teeth need to be removed to prevent the infection from spreading.

All root canalled teeth are dead and harbor infectious microorganisms; so, do all root canalled teeth need to be removed? If you have a root canal and have no significant health problems, *are free from arthritis*, and are in good overall health, it is apparent that your body is capable of protecting you from the infection in the tooth. The tooth can be left alone without any immediate danger. You may be able to live your entire life without complications arising from the tooth. However, as we age our ability to fight off infection decreases, so you will become more susceptible over time.

The absence of symptoms or clearly identifiable signs on X-rays does not prove the absence of infection. All root canalled teeth are infected. The only question is the severity of the infection. If you do have arthritis and, perhaps, other health problems as well, then it is apparent that your body is unable to defend itself against the bacteria in your mouth. You should seriously consider having the root canals removed. Badly diseased teeth also need to be removed.

Extractions have to be done properly. Often after pulling a tooth, the dentist sticks a piece of gauze in the opening to stop the bleeding, and that's about it. However, after the tooth is removed, the socket has to be completely cleaned so that total healing can occur. If tissues, such as torn pieces of ligament or periosteum, are left in the socket, the bone will tend to heal over the top, leaving a hole where new bone cannot form. This hole in the jawbone can persist for the rest of the patient's life and form a site for chronic infection called a *cavitation*. The bone then can become a focus of infection. This condition is easy to prevent by thoroughly cleaning the socket and even removing some of the surrounding bone, if necessary.

Simply removing a bad tooth and cleaning the socket may not be enough. In some cases, the infection has spread from the tooth into the underlying bone. If the infected bone is not removed, it will become a focus of infection. Dr. Price discovered that, in some cases, patients did not recover from systemic health problems after the removal of a badly infected tooth. In most of these cases, the problem was traced back to an infection in the bone surrounding the extracted tooth. Once the infected bone was removed, the patient's health would take a marked turn for the better. So the dentist must examine the jawbone as well and remove all infected tissues.

The removal of root canalled teeth should be done by a dentist who is knowledgeable about the dangers of root canals and cavitations. Many dentists don't understand the danger posed by these situations. The type of dentist you want will proclaim to practice *biological* or *holistic* dentistry.

In some cases, extracting dead and diseased teeth is absolutely necessary if you want to beat arthritis. However, not all diseased teeth need to be extracted. If the infection has not eaten deep into the pulp of the tooth, then there is a possibility that the tooth can be saved. Saving already infected teeth and preventing further infection is essential in combating arthritis. You can accomplish this by an aggressive course of action to improve oral hygiene.

A New Approach to Oral Health

You brush your teeth after every meal, floss, use mouthwash, and visit your dentist every 6 months, as recommended. So, what do you have to worry about? Plenty. Despite good oral hygiene, most people have active decay in their mouths. According to the Centers for Disease Control and Prevention (CDC) website, 90 percent of the population has some level of tooth decay. One third of those over the age of 65 have no natural teeth remaining in their mouths; most all of them lost from disease and infection. Obviously, regular brushing and dental visits have not worked.

Whether you know it or not, chances are you have an infection in your mouth right now. It may not be serious, and there may be no obvious signs that you are aware of.

Signs of infection include chronic bad breath, active cavities, red or swollen gums, gums that bleed easily, receding gums, discolored teeth, pain, sensitivity to heat or cold, loose teeth, and the presence of root canals and possibly crowns as well. If you have any of these conditions, you have a potential problem with bacterial overgrowth. If you are missing teeth (other than wisdom teeth) and have dental fillings or crowns, it indicates that you have had serious problems in the past and likely still do, despite maintaining good oral hygiene.

If regular brushing and flossing isn't effective enough to prevent infection, what can you do? One of the best things you can do to prevent infection and maintain good oral health is to eat a healthy diet. We will discuss this issue in more detail in Chapter 7. Another thing you can do is a technique called *oil pulling*. Oil pulling is an age-old method of oral hygiene that comes to us from Ayurvedic medicine of India. Originally called *oil gargling*, the modern version is referred to as *oil pulling*.

Essentially, oil pulling is rinsing your mouth out with a spoonful of vegetable oil, much like you would do with a mouthwash. The major difference is that you swish the oil in your mouth for 15 to 20 minutes. Although this may sound a bit bizarre, it can work miracles.

What happens when you swish oil in the mouth is that the oil attracts microorganisms and "pulls" them out of the teeth and gums. Mouthwash does not do this. Studies show that oil pulling is more effective at reducing dental plaque (the yellow film that collects on teeth) and gingivitis. In fact, oil pulling is two to seven times more effective at reducing gingivitis than either brushing or using antiseptic mouthwash.[5]

The swishing should be vigorous to work the entire mouth. Don't gargle. Just work it around the teeth and gums. After pulling for 15 to 20 minutes, spit the oil and saliva mixture out. Don't swallow it! It is filled with bacteria, toxins, mucus, and pus.

Oil pulling should be done on an empty stomach. The best time for pulling is first thing in the morning before eating breakfast or brushing your teeth. Oil pulling does not replace your normal brushing and oral hygiene regime; it is something you do in addition to it. Oil pulling should be done every day for the rest of your life, just like brushing. If you have serious health problems or active dental decay, you should oil pull two or three times daily. The best time to do it is before meals.

Oil pulling may stimulate cleansing reactions in the body, such as increasing the drainage of mucus. This is a normal response, so don't be surprised if, during your oil pulling, you feel a need to expel mucus. Spit out the oil, clear your throat and sinuses, take another spoonful of oil, and continue. Keep pulling until you've done it for a total of 15 to 20 minutes. This may sound like a long time, but if you get involved with other tasks such as dressing, making breakfast, reading the newspaper, and such, the time goes by quickly.

When you first start oil pulling, it may feel a little strange swishing oil in your mouth. It takes some people a while to get used to it. But in time, you will feel comfortable, especially if you use a good quality oil.

Any type of vegetable oil will work, but I recommend using coconut oil. The reason for coconut oil is that it has many properties that other oils do not have. Coconut oil has a natural disinfecting nature that can help kill bacteria, viruses, and fungi in the mouth. It also has a soothing and healing effect on the mucous membranes. Other benefits are described in Chapter 6.

Oil pulling is amazingly effective in cleaning infection out of the mouth and reducing the microbial load on the entire body. If an oral infection is chronic and causing systemic problems, then these problems will improve or entirely go away.

Some people are skeptical that a technique as simple as oil pulling can be so effective. The results speak for themselves. One of the first things people notice when they begin oil pulling is better oral health. For example, Lorna describes her experience, "Been oil pulling for two weeks now. Great results! Teeth are tighter, whiter, and cleaner. My entire oral cavity feels as if an entire layer of mucus is removed with each oil pulling. I just feel great all over."

Oil pulling can accomplish more than any other form of oral hygiene. Although oil pulling cannot revive a dead tooth, it can help reduce the infection in that tooth. So if you have root canals that are not seriously infected, oil pulling may keep them from getting worse. Diseased, but living, teeth may be revitalized and saved from extraction or root canalling. Oil pulling saved Amanda from having a root canal. "I have been oil pulling two times a day for about a month now," she says. "I see a very definite improvement. I have had two root canals, and my dentist wanted to do a third. I had severe abscess that caused me constant pain. I started oil pulling and within a few days the pain started to decrease. After a week, I had no pain and the abscess was completely gone. My gums are a healthy pink and they are no longer receding. I had another tooth that was loose and the gums receding badly and needed to be pulled, but the gums have tightened around the tooth and it is no longer loose."

Rhonda, a registered nurse, suffered from multiple oral infections. "My story? It was the teeth and gums. Let me spare you the awful details. Taking care of others did not mean I was wise enough to take care of my own dental health as well as I should have. But within a few days of oil pulling I was out of pain. Within a few weeks I no longer have to have surgery." She says she is going to continue oil pulling for the rest of her life.

Teeth are living tissue and, like other living tissues in the body, have the ability to heal. Even if the teeth are pitted with decay, if the infection is removed and necessary nutrients supplied, the teeth can remineralize. The cavities may not fully fill in, but they can heal over. Teeth cannot heal if infection is present. Oil pulling removes the infection. A mother describes her daughter's experience. "My daughter had *eight* cavities (at the age of five, 16 months ago) that I did not get filled. We started to add more butter and cod liver oil (as recommended by Weston A. Price) and recently we started oil pulling and adding calcium and magnesium. She chipped her front tooth and I took her to the dentist (a different dentist), they did X-rays and came back saying she had only *two* cavities...I looked in her mouth and saw that there was a hole where one of the cavities is...*But* the brown spots (rot) where the cavities were, are *gone!* No brown spots! I am requesting her X-rays from her old dentist to compare them. I think the diet and especially the oil swishing has healed her cavities."

"I started a few months ago," says Tamara. "I've gotten a lot of benefits from it. My three loose teeth are no longer loose. No more sensitive teeth—I can eat hot, cold, etc. without any discomfort to my teeth at all. Severe and repetitive plaque buildup on the inside of my lower front teeth literally fell off in my mouth and has never come back. No more bad breath. Whiter teeth. A tooth that my dentist wanted to give me a root canal on no longer shows any symptoms of being 'dead.' Several cavities were 'gone' when I went to have them filled...Arthritis in my fingers is gone and has never returned. Several chronic pains other than my fingers have also gone away...Honestly, how much better can it get? All these changes, for the cost of a bit of oil."

As oil pulling cleans and heals the mouth, and the entire body responds. Arthritis pain and other health problems apparently related to oral health also improve. "I have been oil pulling for ten days now," says Cherie. "I can't believe how well it works. My teeth look like I just got the best whitening job ever. In addition, my tongue and gums are back to being pink again like when I was younger. In addition to junk that I usually feel is present, somehow in the mouth and teeth feels like it's gone. My energy levels have increased in just ten days. I feel calmer and my mood is good for a change. I had trouble sleeping for years now and I just started going into a deeper more relaxed sleep. My husband just started it because he looked at my teeth and couldn't believe how white they were. Immediately my husband started feeling better and told me his teeth felt clean. Also my husband's pain in his hip has lessened by 50 percent in just three days. I don't know how this stuff works but it's working!"

By pulling the infection out of the teeth, the focus of infection is removed. Without this continual flow of infection into the body, the immune system can sweep up the remaining debris and arthritis symptoms go away. "I have very painful aches in my joints," says Noreen. "I had a hard time standing and my ankles ached horribly while walking. Long story short…I started oil pulling seven days ago and I can hardly believe the results. *My joint pain is almost all gone!* I think I'm still in shock, but I am very grateful and thankful. I oil pull twice a day."

"I thought I was too young to get arthritis," says Linda, "but the joints in my toes, hips, and knees were starting to ache. After two months of oil pulling, all the pain went away. It's been nine months now and the pain has not returned."

If you still have doubts about the effectiveness of oil pulling, I recommend reading my book *Oil Pulling Therapy: Detoxifying and Healing the Body Through Oral Cleansing.* Written in a reader-friendly fashion, this book gives the science behind the therapy and explains how and why oil pulling works. It includes many case studies and success stories from people with a variety of health problems. This book provides powerful convincing evidence for the validity of oil pulling. "Reading this book," says Nona, "has convinced me that oil pulling is a valid therapy to detox the body and especially if there are issues with the mouth, teeth, and gums. I started doing this about a month ago and my arthritis pain is much, much less and my teeth are much whiter; mine have always been a yellow color which made me not want to smile much." Nona has a lot to smile about now.

Aches and pains and other health problems often associated with arthritis also improve. "It worked wonders for my fibromyalgia pain," says Beth. "I oil pull for 15 minutes a day. I also have TMJ and didn't think I would be able to do this for that length of time because of the pain in my jaw. But after just a couple of minutes of swishing, my jaw pain left. The stiffness, pain, and soreness in my entire body is gone! I have been suffering from fibromyalgia for over 15 years and this is the only thing I have tried that has given me relief."

"I began oil pulling eight months ago," says Sonya. "I suffered with chronic fatigue and fibromyalgia for over 12 years. I had chronic pain so bad that it hurt to move. Walking was difficult. I ended up spending most of my time in bed. I started oil pulling and changes occurred gradually week after week, until my health was back to normal. Oil pulling literally saved my life!"

Oil pulling is inexpensive and totally benign. It has no side effects nor does it interfere with any medications or diets. You don't even swallow the oil, so you are not ingesting anything. It is a very simple procedure with a very powerful healing effect.

While oil pulling is very useful, it is only one step in the Seven Step Arthritis Battle Plan described in this book. The following chapters describe the remaining six steps.

Chapter 6

Nature's Antibiotic

A Natural Defense Against Infection

Oil pulling will help draw the infection out of the mouth, but what about infections in other parts of the body? You need something that can kill a systemic infection. Antibiotics may work, if you have a bacterial infection. But if you have a viral or fungal infection or an infection from drug-resistant bacteria, antibiotics won't do any good. Besides, you probably won't be able to find a doctor who will prescribe antibiotics without a good reason, and chronic arthritis usually isn't a good enough reason for them.

What you need is a potent, nonprescription, all-purpose, antibiotic, antiviral, antifungal remedy that is completely safe to consume and has no adverse side effects, even if taken for extended periods of time. That eliminates all prescription and over-the-counter drugs.

What is needed is something that is completely safe to eat—like food. Not just any food. Not all so-called "foods" are fit to eat. We need a natural, wholesome food that offers all of the above characteristics. One such food comes readily to mind: coconut! And more specifically, coconut oil.

You may ask, why coconut oil? While there are other foods that offer some antibiotic-like properties, none are as potent or as effective, yet as safe, as coconut oil. Coconut oil has a long history of effective use against infections, with an extensive accumulation of documented studies to back it up. It is, in fact, one of nature's finest antibiotic foods.

Coconut oil is considered a *functional food* because it has health benefits beyond those provided by its nutritional content. Functional foods have therapeutic value that can protect us from various health problems. One of the many functions that coconut oil provides is protection against infection. I have seen it clear up flu symptoms almost overnight, stop bladder infections, heal chronic skin and nail fungus infections, bring quick relief from Crohn's disease, quench herpes infections, restore energy in those with chronic fatigue, and bring relief to chronic arthritis sufferers, among others. Medical researchers are now using it in the fight against difficult-to-treat conditions such as hepatitis C and AIDS.

Many people have been using coconut oil successfully to fight a variety of infectious conditions. While in the hospital for tests on a blood condition, Glenn picked up an infection and developed a severe case of prostatitis. Prostatitis is inflammation of the prostate gland—an organ about the size and shape of a walnut, located just below the bladder in males. Infection is the most common cause and can be acute or chronic.

To fight the infection, doctors started Glenn on antibiotic therapy, first with Cipro and then with Bactrim. "Cipro gave me terrible headaches and a case of the handshakes as well as a nasty case of drug-induced rosacea," recalls Glenn. "Worse, after all this, it didn't relieve the problems. Next, I tried Bactrim. I got a terrible rash and the drug-induced rosacea got even worse. I was at a loss and getting worse by the week. Finally my urologist told me to tough it out. It would eventually burn out. Knowing that chronic inflammation also can lead to cancer, I wasn't to keen to allow my prostate gland to be infected for the next 10 years."

A few days later, while doing some research on the Internet, Glenn found that candida can be a prime cause of prostatitis. Candida is a fungus, not a bacterium. No wonder the antibiotics hadn't worked. He also learned that coconut oil has remarkable antibacterial, antifungal, and anti-candida properties. "This interested me," says Glenn. "The website referenced a guy by the name of Bruce Fife who is a leading authority on coconut oil. I read his book (*Coconut Cures: Preventing and Treating Common Health Problems with Coconut*) and it seems that the therapeutic dose of coconut oil is 4 tablespoons per day for as long as it takes to rid yourself of your problem…So I bought a tub of the stuff and started taking it. For the first three days after I started taking it I had what can only be described as a healing reaction. All my symptoms were much worse. Then on day four, I started to get relief. And within 30 days I was almost symptom free."

That wasn't all. In addition to getting rid of the infection, the coconut oil had some other remarkable benefits. "I have *much* more energy," exclaims Glenn, "my skin is smoother and nicer and I have lost about 10 pounds. And, oh yeah, the rosacea is *gone!* I have started to use the stuff topically for thick toenails and athlete's foot and those maladies are on their way out also. After only a few weeks of topical treatment, my toenails are regrowing normally and my athlete's foot is a fading memory."

What makes coconut oil such an effective antimicrobial agent? And what makes coconut oil different from any other dietary fat? The key to unlocking the secret to coconut oil's remarkable healing powers comes from the study of human breast milk.

Years ago it was discovered that human breast milk contains a unique group of saturated fats known as medium-chain triglycerides (MCTs). These fats are very different from the fats found in meats and vegetables.

When eaten, the body transforms MCTs into monoglycerides and medium-chain fatty acids (MCFAs), both of which possess powerful antimicrobial properties capable of killing disease-causing bacteria, viruses, and fungi.[1] It is primarily the presence of MCTs in human breast milk that protects babies from infections for the first few months of their lives, while their immune systems are still developing.[2] MCFAs from MCTs are nature's antimicrobials. They are in mother's milk to protect newborn infants from disease. Although deadly to disease-causing germs, they are completely harmless to us.

What does this have to do with coconut oil? Like mother's milk, coconut oil also contains MCTs. In fact, coconut oil is composed predominantly of MCTs. The MCTs in coconut oil are identical to those found in mother's milk and possess the same antimicrobial potential. For this reason, food manufacturers have been putting coconut oil, or MCTs derived from coconut oil, into baby formula for years in order

Triglyceride

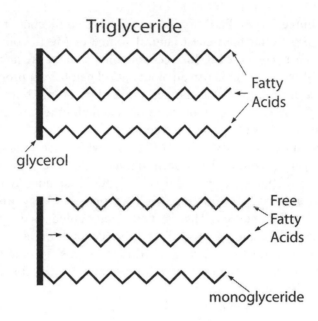

Triglycerides are composed of three fatty acid molecules joined together by a glycerol molecule. Digestive enzymes break the bonds between the fatty acids and the glycerol molecules producing free fatty acids and monoglycerides.

to give the formula the same disease-fighting capability as natural breast milk.[3] If you fed your children formula when they were infants, you were giving them coconut oil in some form or another.

In the realm of dietary fats and oils, MCTs are unique. Most of the fats in our food are composed almost entirely of what is known as long-chain triglycerides (LCTs). These long-chain triglycerides are molecular structures that have a long chain of carbon atoms serving as the backbone of the fat molecule. In contrast, MCTs, as the name implies, are molecular structures that have a shorter carbon backbone. This difference in size makes all the difference in the world and gives MCTs unique physical and biological properties.

About 98 to 100 percent of the fats and oils you eat every day consist of LCTs. Other than breast milk, there are very few good dietary sources of MCTs. Dairy butter and whole milk contain a small amount. But by far the richest natural source of MCTs comes from coconut. There are more MCTs in coconut oil than there are in mother's milk, a lot more. For this reason, coconut oil can have a pronounced impact on our health, just as mother's milk does on newborn infants. This is what makes coconut oil different from all other oils and what gives it much of its unique healing character.

Medium-chain fatty acids (MCFAs), which are created from MCTs during digestion, have been studied extensively as potential antimicrobial agents that can be used in foods, cosmetics, and drugs. Researchers have found that MCFAs possess very powerful antimicrobial properties. This is well documented in the medical literature. Studies show that MCFAs, from coconut oil, are effective in killing bacteria that cause such things as gastric ulcers, sinus infections, bladder infections, gum disease and cavities, pneumonia, gonorrhea, and many other illnesses.[4-9]

They kill fungi and yeasts that cause ringworm, athlete's foot, jock itch, and candidiasis.[10-12]

They kill viruses that cause influenza, measles, herpes, mononucleosis, and hepatitis C.[13-17] They are so potent that they even kill HIV—the AIDS virus.[18-20]

There are numerous published studies and even entire books describing the antimicrobial effects of MCFAs derived from coconut oil.[21] Most of the studies have been done in laboratory settings. The evidence is clear; MCFAs do kill disease-causing bacteria, viruses, and fungi in experimental situations in the laboratory. But what about in the real world? Can consuming coconut oil provide the same protection? The evidence says yes. Clinical studies and case histories do show that simply consuming coconut oil can have a beneficial effect against infectious illnesses.

Because of the published studies that have shown that MCFAs kill the AIDS virus, many HIV-infected people have added coconut to their treatment programs with success. For example, Chris Dafoe of Cloverdale, Indiana, had a viral load of 600,000, which indicated the infection was rapidly overpowering his body. He began eating coconut every day. Within weeks his viral load dropped to undetectable

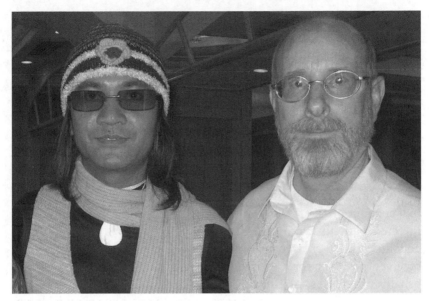

The author (right) with Tony V. (left).

levels.[22] Many other HIV-infected individuals have reported similar experiences.

In another case, Tony V. was diagnosed with full-blown AIDS. AIDS attacks the immune system of its victims, thus increasing their vulnerability to other infections. In fact, AIDS patients usually die from secondary infections rather than from the AIDS virus itself. Tony was in terrible shape. His immune system was so weakened that he was riddled with secondary infections. He had lost a substantial amount of weight, suffered with chronic pneumonia, struggled with chronic fatigue, experienced repeated bouts of nausea and diarrhea, had oral candidiasis, and was covered from head to foot with skin infections. His skin was an angry red, cracking, flaking, and weeping. His skin was so bad that the hair on his head was falling out in clumps. He wore a wig to hide the bald spots and oozing sores. He was so far gone that his doctors told him he had only a matter of months to live.

Unable to work because of his illness, he had little money and could not afford to continue to buy medication. He asked the government for help. He was referred to a doctor who just happened to have published some studies on the therapeutic effects of coconut oil. He told Tony to consume 6 tablespoons of coconut oil daily, along with rubbing more oil on the lesions all over his body. Tony began doing as he was directed. To the surprise of his other doctors, nine months later Tony was still alive. Not only was he alive, but he was thriving. The coconut oil healed him from all of his secondary infections and brought the HIV under control. He regained his lost weight, his hair grew back, and his skin was clear and healthy, with no sign of infection.[23] It has been four years now and Tony is still doing well.

A clinical study carried out in the Philippines provided more proof that coconut oil is effective in fighting off infection. A group of HIV infected patients were given the equivalent of 3½ tablespoons of coconut oil a day. Because of their poor financial situation, they received no other form of treatment. Without treatment, the disease usually progresses, and health slowly declines. However, with just coconut oil, after six months 60 percent of the patients showed lower viral levels and improved health status.[24]

Studies by Gilda Erguiza, MD, and colleagues have shown that coconut oil added to standard antibiotic therapy improves recovery from community-acquired pneumonia. Community-acquired pneumonia is an infection of the lungs that is contracted outside a hospital setting. It is a serious infection in children. In a presentation delivered to the American College of Chest Physicians in Philadelphia, Dr. Erguiza described her findings.[25] The study included 40 children between the ages of three months to five years, all suffering from community-acquired pneumonia and treated intravenously with the antibiotic ampicillin. Half of the group was also given a daily dose of coconut oil at 2 ml per kilogram of body weight. The oil was given for three days in a row. The researchers found that the respiratory rate normalized in 32.6 hours for the coconut oil group versus 48.2 hours for the control group. After three days, patients in the control group were more likely than those in the coconut oil group to still have wheezing in the lungs—60 percent of the controls still had wheezing compared to only 25 percent of the coconut oil group. Those in the coconut oil group also recovered from their fevers quicker, had normal oxygen saturation faster, and had shorter hospital stays.

What People Are Saying About Coconut Oil

Thousands of people are currently using coconut oil as a home-remedy against infections with good success. Some people prefer to use *virgin* coconut oil over ordinary coconut oil. The term "virgin" indicates that the oil that has undergone minimal processing so it retains all of its natural nutrients and flavor. Both forms of coconut oil have been used successfully.

For example, Pix states, "I went to an OBGYN. I had a pap-smear and the result was BV (bacterial vaginosis). I went through meds (Flagyl) for 7 days. Discharge was okay but the itch is still there. I went to the same OB again, she prescribed Canesten vaginal tablet. It didn't work!!! I was really going out my mind to find a solution to my problem. A client referred me to another OB, Dr. Myrna Habaña at VRP Hospital. She did an exam and could see nothing wrong except for the coarse hair (pubes), she prescribed Travocort cream and virgin coconut oil (VCO). My god, first night I applied both, I couldn't believe it! The first decent sleep of the year! No itch!...and it doesn't sting anymore. I can live normally, sleep normally. VCO calmed my irritated skin."

Melissa E. says, "I found myself leafing through Bruce Fife's book just before Christmas, and was so fascinated that I walked out having bought the book and a jar of organic unrefined coconut oil. Immediately I started using it on my skin and added a small amount to my diet. On New Year's Eve I felt the onslaught of the flu....scratchy throat and fatigue....so I added more coconut oil to a soup I was making (to which I also added fresh ginger and reishi mushroom and garlic). Overnight the symptoms progressed to my lungs...a deep cough signifying bronchitis. I had more coconut oil, probably 3 or 4 tablespoons. Usually when my body is successfully fighting an illness like this, the symptoms gradually subside over a couple of days at best. But in this case, by nightfall of New Years day, *all* my symptoms were absolutely *gone!* Wow. I could only imagine those fatty acids busting up all the influenza viruses one by one as the reason. I have never experienced such a quick and complete turnaround."

Mike says, "I wanted to thank you for enlightening me to the benefits of coconut oil. I am 29 years old and have been suffering with ulcerative colitis for 14 years. My father had ulcerative colitis that went untreated and led to cancer and his death at the age of 46, so I have always been aware of the seriousness. I never experienced coconut oil until my wife found your cookbooks! I visited your website and ordered your *Coconut Cures* book and was blown away page after page. In addition to colitis, I have several other medical problems that were treated with coconut oil so how can I not give it a shot.

"I built up to a maintenance level of 1-2 tablespoons in my coffee every morning and started feeling better after about 1 month. Nine months later I had my yearly colonoscopy check up (required for colitis patients of any age) and my doctor was shocked! Not only has the disease reversed itself, none of the biopsies revealed any indication of colitis and I essentially have a normal person's colon!! I told him about coconut oil and, of course, my doctor thought that the medication was cause for improvement but said to definitely keep doing whatever I'm doing. If only my father had this knowledge when my father was young, he could have seen his kids grow up."

"I've had chronic bladder infections for twenty years," says Cindy D. "I've been to numerous doctors with no positive results and most of the time I was worse. After the last doctor I swore I would not go to another doctor unless I was dying and had no choice. I began to research natural remedies. I tried so many things it would be hard to list. They helped to some extent but didn't cure my infections. I found your website and tried coconut oil. In one month's time I have not had one bladder infection. I'm taking one tablespoon 3 times a day with meals. I've put the oil on cuts and healed so quickly I couldn't believe it. My husband eats popcorn every night and I started using coconut oil instead of canola oil. He loves the flavor of the popcorn. I'm anxious to see what other benefits we'll get by using the oil long term."

Holistic minded medical doctors, nurses, and nutritionists are also using coconut oil and recommending it to their patients. Dr. Eliza Perez Francisco, MD says, "In my clinical practice at St. Luke's Medical Center, I use virgin coconut oil for the elderly in relation to physiologic changes that occur with aging. Virgin coconut oil can address sensory losses, tooth and gum problems, changes in the intestinal tract, changes in the immune system, changes in body composition, and changes that come with menopause and andropause...A combination of old age and malnutrition makes older people vulnerable to pneumonia, UTI, and bedsores. Virgin coconut oil can help fight infection in the early stages. Take the case of a 76-year-old who developed painful herpes zoster on his trunk. The antibiotic cream given to him only lasted for one application because the area affected was so wide. But when virgin coconut oil was applied all over the skin for a week, the patient reported relief from itch and the lesions dried up."

Dr. S. Kumar, MD, states, "I am a primary care practitioner or general practitioner with priority in nutritional medicine as the healing component. I have read Dr. Fife's, Dr. Dayrit's, and Prof. Mary G. Enig's books and am using only virgin coconut oil (VCO) for cooking and also orally when down with the flu, etc. I strongly advise my patients to consume more VCO when sick and advocate to all ages from newborns to the old and sick, including those with diabetic, hypertensive, heart, and skin ailments and even those stricken with cancer. Over the last two years I've seen patients get better. It is difficult sometimes for some patients initially to accept VCO. They think I am going 'nuts'! The truth is being revealed and allopathic medicine has to admit all this while they have been wrong and it is still not too late to rectify this mistake. I still get criticisms from many, but I believe in due time the critics will be silenced."

MCFAs Versus Drugs

For acute bacterial infections, antibiotics are useful. However, antibiotic therapy isn't without risks. While antibiotics may be necessary at times, the problem with them is that they are often toxic to us as well as to the bacteria they are designed to kill. Side effects include nausea, diarrhea, colitis, kidney dysfunction, liver damage, blood disorders, deafness, and increased sensitivity to the sun, to mention just a few.

In contrast, coconut oil does no harm. It has no adverse side effects, except that it might cause a die-off reaction, that is, it will kill so many harmful microbes that the body may experience a short period of discomfort as the dead organisms and toxins are expelled. While this cleansing reaction may feel uncomfortable for a day to two, it is not harmful but is a sign of healing and improving health.

Placebo or Cure?

Many people can give testimony to the success of coconut oil in overcoming infections and other health problems. Some critics might claim that these remarkable recoveries are merely the result of the placebo effect. In other words, it was all in their minds. They *believed* they would get better using the oil and so they did. It was just a psychological effect. The problem with this argument is that even animals, who are not influenced by belief, get better when given coconut oil, as the following account illustrates.

"About a week after we moved in to our new home, our eight-year old dog, Davis got deathly ill. We actually thought he may have broken his back on the stairs. He could not walk and had to be carried everywhere. The vet was certain that he had hurt his back as well, but on the second day, he started having blisters on his feet and on the back of his body. When he stood up on his feet, they would just bleed. (Just lovely in the new house!!!) After inconclusive tests, as well as even a spinal tap, they decided to call it an autoimmune disease. Still not sure quite the diagnosis, but he was on death's bed. After $1,500 in tests and medications, the vet still was unsure of the prognosis and suggested to put him out of his misery. Davis was still unable to walk, but now unable to open one eye and had large half-dollar size lesions all over his back and hind legs.

"After making the appointment on Friday, to put him to sleep on Monday, I decided to try one last thing over the weekend. I read on the Internet about coconut oil being good for dog's immune system. Desperately I tried it, and miraculously about four hours after his first dose, he got up and walked. Within a day, his feet stopped bleeding and he was once again walking over to the food bowl! I am convinced and just amazed! Funny how after $1,500 of tests and meds from the vet, a $15 jar of coconut oil healed him!!! It has now been two weeks and he is back to normal."

Drugs affect our health in other ways, too. Antibiotics kill *all* the bacteria in the body, including "friendly" gut bacteria. In the absence of the friendly bacteria in the intestinal tract, candida, a troublesome yeast, is allowed to grow unrestrained. This often leads to candidiasis. Some "unfriendly" drug resistant, toxin-producing bacteria, such as *Clostridium difficile*, are also allowed to proliferate, causing a shift in the types of microbes that live in the gut, which can lead to digestive troubles.

Unlike antibiotics, MCFAs do not kill all bacteria. They are more selective. They kill harmful bacteria but leave the good bacteria alone. An added benefit with MCFAs is that they also kill candida. So the microbial environment within the intestinal tract improves with the use of coconut oil.

Candida is the most common fungus that causes ill health in humans. There are many species of candida. *Candida albicans* is the most notorious. It is the primary cause of vaginal yeast infections, systemic yeast infections (candidiasis), oral yeast infections (thrush), and skin infections (diaper rash and skin fungus). It is also known to attack the joints and cause arthritis. While not the most deadly fungus, it is the most troublesome. Part of the reason is because it is a normal inhabitant of the digestive tract. We have candida living with us constantly. It usually causes little problem unless we have other health issues. Candida is an opportunistic organism. It pretty much behaves itself as long as we take care of ourselves and are healthy. But if we become sick, eat poorly, or take medications, especially antibiotics, it grabs the opportunity and can quickly multiply out of control.

Coconut oil, taken internally with food or as a medicine, can stop candida and put it back in its place. In a study published in the *Journal of Medicinal Food*, researchers collected 52 clinical specimens of different species of candida, comprising 17 samples of *Candida albicans*, 9 *Candida glabrata*, 7 *Candida tropicalis*, 7 *Candida parapsilosis*, 6 *Candida stellatoidea*, and 6 *Candida krusel*.[26] The effectiveness of virgin coconut oil as an antifungal agent was evaluated on each species and compared to fluconazole—a commercial fungicide. Coconut oil killed all the species of candida and was just as effective as fluconazole, if not better. Out of all the species, coconut oil was most effective against *Candida albicans,* displaying twice

Herpes Simplex Virus

For 24 years I have battled herpes simplex type II (not type I) both genitally and in my mouth, and on my nose. My infection is not the typical type where you get some blisters that heal. I have always had a severe systemic type reaction whenever I get an outbreak which at times for many years was as frequent as twice a month, barely healed and I would come down with it again. But the worst part is that prior to the outbreak I would suffer extreme fatigue and very nasty headaches that feel like a chainsaw is ripping into my brain, whether I had the genital or facial blisters. It affected my ability to think and my memory and I worried that the virus was eating away at my brain. I used Acyclovir preventively for three years to fairly good effect, until it stopped working altogether. Needless to say herpes has been an incredibly destructive force in my life, not to mention the emotional trauma and effect on my sex life and relationships.

I've also had such severe prostatitis that I couldn't pee for days and although my Dr. says it's not a cause of prostatitis I'm almost certain that mine is caused by herpes. None of the antibiotics she's given me have helped it.

Since the antivirals no longer work (I've tried the others) I have for years restricted my chocolate intake and nuts as these are two of the highest sources of arginine which the virus needs to trigger and sustain an infection, though there are lower levels in a lot of common foods that are hard to avoid. I have also used sterolins for many years to suppress outbreaks and they help quite a bit, but neither completely stops outbreaks.

Around Christmas (maybe 10 days into my coconut regime) I became reckless and consumed some chocolate and nuts. I was surprised and happy that it didn't trigger an outbreak, and it was then I started looking into the effects of coconut oil. Wow, I found out it has an anti-herpes effect. Could it really be preventing my outbreaks? Previously I could guarantee an infection if I overdid it on the chocolate or nuts, so I decided to have some more chocolate, peanut butter and real fresh coconut which also contains high levels of arginine, and which I had been avoiding for that reason. Still no infection. I was amazed and decided to eat chocolate and peanut butter freely whenever I wanted. Still no herpes infections. To say that I am amazed is certainly an understatement considering the hell I've been suffering for 24 years.

Shortly after Christmas I noticed my constipation was gone altogether. The only thing that was different was the coconut oil.

Last week, about 5 or 6 weeks into the coconut oil I started noticing no prostate symptoms. It's only been a week since then so it's hard to say my prostatitis is cured but considering my track record on coconut oil 44 years of constipation and 24 years of severe herpes eliminated, I'm hopeful that it will be the same with the prostatitis.

I'm extremely happy to have found coconut oil.

—David

the killing power of fluconazole. Coconut oil, therefore, is potentially more effective in fighting candida than the drug fluconazole, which is sold under the trade names Diflucan and Trican. Side effects to fluconazole include rash, nausea, vomiting, diarrhea, headache, fatigue, anorexia, blood disorders, seizures, and liver failure. Coconut oil, on the other hand, is completely non-toxic.

Antibiotics have been hailed as the miracle drugs of the twentieth century. At first they seemed to be effective in stopping many of the dreaded diseases of the past. However, new strains of bacteria have been arising that are resistant to these drugs, and infectious illnesses are on the rise. The overuse of antibiotics has led to the increase of these so-called supergerms that are immune to antibiotics. Scientists are continually trying to develop new antibiotics to fight these new drug-resistant strains of bacteria.

Drug-resistant bacteria, however, are not immune to the action of MCFAs. MCFAs kill these sugergerms just as easily as if they were ordinary bacteria.[27] Fungi can also develop drug resistance, but MCFAs kill them as well.[28]

In addition, MCFAs do not promote antibiotic resistance or the development of supergerms. When MCFAs come into contact with microorganisms, these fatty acids are absorbed into the fatty outer membranes of these organisms, which decreases the strength of the membrane wall to such a degree that the germs simply fall apart and die. White blood cells then clean up the debris. It is believed to be unlikely for organisms to evolve or mutate to overcome this particular killing action. So, MCFAs are just as effective against drug-resistant organisms as they are against regular ones.

MCFAs do another thing antibiotics can't; they kill viruses. Antibiotics can't touch viruses. In fact, there are no medications that can effectively kill viruses. Vaccination is the only weapon we have against them. When you get the flu there isn't anything the doctor can do for you. All he can do is give you medications that may make the symptoms easier to cope with, but your body has to do all the work in fighting off the infection. Some viral infections can linger in the body indefinitely. Once infected with herpes or hepatitis C, for example, you have it for life. MCFAs offer a natural, harmless method of ridding the body of these troublemakers, or at least of allowing you to live a normal life without serious symptoms. No medication can do that. MCFAs apparently can also pass through the blood-brain barrier and reach into places many drugs can't, clearing out deep seated infections. Coconut oil is perhaps the strongest antibacterial, antiviral, and antifungal aid you can get without a doctor's prescription.

Although MCFAs are deadly to many disease-causing microorganisms, they are completely harmless to us. In fact, they are so safe that nature puts them into mother's milk to nourish newborn infants.

As safe and as good as they are, MCFAs do not kill *all* harmful microorganisms. Consequently, some disease-causing organisms are unaffected. For example, rhinovirus, which causes the common cold, and hepatitis A virus are two such organisms.

If coconut oil is so effective, why haven't we heard more about it in the treatment of infectious illnesses? The problem with coconut oil is that it is a natural product. Pharmaceutical companies cannot patent it, so they have little interest in developing or promoting it. Most of the interest has come from the health food and supplement industry. In fact, coconut oil in one form or another has been used for some time. Caprylic acid, one of the MCFAs in coconut oil, is a popular ingredient in many anti-candida formulations. Monolaurin, another coconut oil derived supplement, is used as a general-purpose antibiotic. Fractionated coconut oil, also known as MCT oil, is a common ingredient in many health and fitness products. Coconut oil has even been put into gel capsules as a dietary supplement. Of course, you can also find pure coconut oil in just about any health food store.

Coconut Oil and Arthritis

The good news about coconut oil for arthritis sufferers is that many of the microorganisms that are killed by MCFAs are also associated with arthritis. That means that consuming coconut oil on a regular basis may be useful in helping to relieve the symptoms of infectious arthritis.

I've written several books on the health benefits of coconut. Many readers have contacted me and have described how coconut oil has helped them overcome various health problems. One of the conditions that readers frequently mention is arthritis. At first, I didn't know what to make of it. I didn't know exactly how the oil was affecting the joints. But apparently it was, because so many people were experiencing improvement. Later, as I began to study focal infections, I discovered the cause of arthritis and then realized why coconut oil is so beneficial for this condition. The antimicrobial effect of the MCFAs in the oil reduces the systemic infection, which in turn reduces infection in the joints. Combined with the body's immune defenses, the infection comes under control. For many people, simply taking coconut oil daily was enough to completely rid themselves of joint pain. Others experienced dramatic improvement. Even a partial improvement is welcome.

Rudy, 52, suffered from gouty arthritis. Many parts of his body ached, but mostly his right arm and shoulder, which caused "irritating pain." He was taking allopurinol to inhibit uric acid production, with little apparent benefit. Friends told him about coconut oil. He thought

"Why not try it?" so he did. He began eating two spoonfuls with lunch and two with dinner, usually pouring it over whatever he was eating. "After a week," he says, "I noticed my right arm moving more freely, and the pain subsiding. After a month the pain was gone!"

Annette R. suffered from arthritis and back problems. She began using coconut oil and noticed results within three weeks. "I used to have a problem just getting up out of my seat," she says. "Since I have been using coconut oil, I just get right up with no problems. I thought I had to get a new mattress because my back was hurting so bad, but now I have no problems. (I am still going to get a new mattress anyway.) I just want to say that I am sold on this coconut oil and have recommended it to family and friends, and they are having great results from it."

Belinda R. is amazed at what coconut oil has done for her husband: "My husband has regained complete use of his shoulders and his joints are pain free for the first time in over 12 years! He takes about 1-2 tablespoons of coconut oil in his coffee every morning. He has lost 15 pounds and noticed an increase in energy the *first* day he took the coconut oil."

"I'm a 49-year-old lady with already one knee replacement and creaky joints," says Beth. "There is a great difference in my joints from taking virgin coconut oil daily, like I'm internally lubricated! The improvement is dramatic."

Bobbie B. purchased her first gallon of coconut oil over the Internet. "Our lives have never been the same since," she says. "We immediately loved the fine, rich and creamy texture of the VCO. Then the taste blew us away. Very mild coconut flavor with a texture of pure heaven. Knowing how healthy it is to eat totally enhances the experience of virgin coconut oil!!! Imagine something akin to a yummy, creamy truffle that actually enhances your health! I eat a tablespoon straight twice a day and use it exclusively for all cooking needs!!! I used to be an olive oil only person. Now olive oil is reserved for salad dressing. Before the VCO, I was suffering from arthritis in my hips, knees, and feet. I had various dry skin conditions that were a constant battle. I was at least 30 pounds heavier. I changed nothing in the way that I eat, having a pretty healthy diet as a vegetarian. My skin conditions cleared up within two weeks of use. My skin took on a much more youthful appearance. Friends who hadn't seen me for a while would remark on the overall improvement in my skin, my weight, my hair and my energy level! I began to feel more lubricated in the joints and the arthritis faded into the background and is hardly there now."

"For about a couple of years now," says Conrad, "I've had a stiff neck and saw a doctor about it some time ago. He said it was a mild case of arthritis, aggravated by my work, which compels me to sit in front of a computer for long hours every day. At one point, I was having problems twisting my neck to look behind me when turning to my right while driving. For Christmas I received a couple of bottles of coconut oil. I took no notice of it, having been a veteran tester of various herbal products that purported to ease or even cure my gout. That has included things from cherry extracts to alfalfa sprouts. None of it did the wonders they promised. So my gift lay unappreciated in the back of the cupboard. The following year at a party some people got to talking about the benefits of coconut oil. A couple swore to its efficiency. I mentioned that I had gotten it as a present last Christmas, but hadn't touched it. They eagerly pressed me into trying it. What had I got to lose? they asked. I decided to try it, not least so I'd have something to report to them next time they interrogated me. I started taking the stuff a little more than three months ago. The label on the bottle said three tablespoons a day, but I took two. The stiffness in my neck wondrously disappeared for the most part. I do still experience some stiffness in my neck now and then, but that is more the exception than the rule. Although it hasn't cured my gout yet, it has made walking much easier, something I've been at pains to do for some time now, my left knee in particular having become stiff. On the whole, I've never felt quite better."

Even medical doctors are beginning to take notice. Arlene Bourne, MD, said, "I purchased your book on coconut oil a month ago and since then have experienced significant pain relief from seronegative arthritis. It's *real!* I've taken it upon myself to mention it to each patient I see and anyone I interact with. I direct them to your website and also caution that they should accept the information from the people who actually research coconut rather than any other uninvolved source. Thanks a million."

Fibromyalgia sufferers also benefit. Dr. R. L. Meliodon, DC, says, I have been a chronic fatigue/fibromyalgia sufferer for the past six years. I never missed a day's work because of it or anything else. I just pulled myself up by the bootstraps and hoped I could make it through another day. The past year got me so worn-out that I eventually had no other choice than to shorten my workday from 12 hours to eight. Even eight hours was a killer. I tried many things over the years to deal with the CF/FM but never found anything of lasting value until I stumbled upon coconut oil."

Dr. Meliodon discovered coconut oil on the Internet when he did a search for "fibromyalgia cure." "I immediately found three or four of the first listings to mention something about coconut oil and I didn't think much about it or give it much credence…after all what could coconut oil possibly do for my fibromyalgia? But it was a blogger's comment that really hit home…it simply said. 'I took coconut oil for my fibromyalgia…my pain is gone, my pain is gone, my pain is gone!' I immediately ran out to my nearest health food store and bought a bottle. I haven't been the same since! My pain is gone, gone, gone, too. At least 70 percent of it! I can now work the 12 hours a day again."

Coconut oil can be helpful in relieving the pain of arthritis and fibromyalgia, however, it should not be considered a complete cure unless it removes the source of the infection. In most cases, that source will be in the mouth. Simply eating the oil is not enough to kill oral infections. Good oral hygiene combined with oil pulling will pull infection out of the mouth. Taking coconut internally will rid it from the body. These steps, plus the other five steps in the Arthritis Battle Plan, should be taken for complete success.

Even after joint pain has gone, incorporating coconut oil into your daily diet is an excellent way to stay healthy. If you are fighting an active infection, I recommend taking 3 to 4 tablespoons a day. Once the infection is under control, a good maintenance dose is 1 to 3 tablespoons daily.

Chapter 7

The Anti-Arthritis Diet

"After exercising one day I noticed that my right big toe was intensely painful and slightly swollen," says Michael, a 55-year-old computer technician. "Since there was no pain before my workout I assumed that I must have done something to have sprained it. I took it easy for a few weeks to let it heal, but the pain never went away. I am fortunate enough to live in an arca where there are many hiking trails and I like to hike. I would hike my usual 4 or 5 miles and have to limp home in pain. I gave up hiking. I could barely walk without pain. Running or aerobics intensified the pain. I even stopped all exercise for several weeks hoping it might help. But it didn't. Nothing I did could relieve the pain. If I didn't move the toe at all it didn't bother me, so with my desk job I could get by, but as soon as I moved it or walked the pain made itself known. For the next 4 to 5 months the pain didn't let up. Although I thought I was immune to arthritis because of my healthy lifestyle, I now realized it was a reality.

"I had about 10 pounds I wanted to lose so I started on a low-carbohydrate diet, eating only fresh whole foods. I eliminated all sweets, breads, and grains. I rarely eat junk foods. I eat mostly organic. After about a week I noticed something wonderful—the pain in my foot was starting to lessen. After three weeks the pain that had plagued me for months was essentially gone, along with the 10 pounds I wanted to lose. I couldn't believe that cutting carbs out of my diet would have such an effect. I've since added some good carbs back into my diet, and six months later the pain is still gone."

Does diet affect arthritis? You bet it does! Diet is the single most important factor influencing arthritis. Your diet can be the cause of arthritis or the cure.

Back in the early 1980s, health writer Norman Ford developed an interest in arthritis and began interviewing people with the disease. He spoke with hundreds of arthritis sufferers and discovered that about 10 percent had experienced a spontaneous remission without a relapse. He questioned these people further to discover what they had done that could have led to their recovery. Most all of them had gone though the normal course of drug therapy without relief or improvement. The one thing they all had in common was that they, either by design or by chance, had made radical changes in their living habits just prior to recovery. Some cut out smoking or alcohol, but far more reported having made major changes in their eating habits, usually switching to a diet of fresh, whole foods.[1]

Do Food Allergies Cause Arthritis?

Many years ago it was discovered that diet plays an important role in the development and the cure of arthritis, in particular rheumatoid and gouty arthritis, but also osteoarthritis. When arthritis patients were put on therapeutic fasts of 7-10 days or more, their pains went away. Obviously, something associated with food was affecting the joints. Simply eliminating all foods brought substantial improvement. However, fasting therapy wasn't the solution. It only brought temporary relief. When normal eating was resumed, the pain came back.

This effect led doctors to believe that perhaps arthritis was caused by a food allergy. Simply removing the allergen (food that triggers an allergy) from the diet could, doctors hoped, cure the disease. This idea has become very popular, and many arthritis sufferers claim that removing allergens from their diets helps them.

The foods that most often cause allergies are wheat, soy, nuts, eggs, milk, peanuts, chicken, fish, and shellfish, but almost any food can be at fault. The solanaceae family of flowering plants has been particularly targeted as a possible source of arthritis-causing foods, but not because they cause allergies, but rather, they are believed to be inherently unhealthful, even toxic. Commonly known as the nightshade family or potato family, the solanaceae group of vegetables includes white potatoes, tomatoes, bell peppers, chili peppers, eggplant, and paprika.

The campaign against nightshades was started in the late 1970s by Norman F. Childers, a horticulturist. When he was in his early 50s, he began to experience "achy, hurting knees and ankle joints." He removed potatoes, eggplant, and other solanaceae vegetables from his diet and the problem disappeared. Impressed by the results he wrote a book claiming that vegetables in the nightshade family are toxic and cause arthritis as well as heart aliments, high blood pressure, stroke, cancer, Alzheimer's disease, premature aging, and an overall degeneration of health. You might keep in mind that Childers' field of expertise is plant cultivation, not medicine. Despite a complete lack of scientific evidence to back him up, many people still believe in his theory.

Medical research has found no correlation between these foods and arthritis or any other ailments. In fact, members of this family are very nutritious and are actually used as medicine to help *relieve* arthritis symptoms. One such medication is a cream containing capsaicin, the ingredient in chili peppers that makes them "hot." Studies show that this spicy ingredient is beneficial in that it calms inflammation and sooths irritation.[2] Arthritis patients report reduced pain and greater mobility in affected joints. So, instead of causing arthritis, this hot pepper extract eases the symptoms without adverse effects.

Over the years, hundreds of studies have examined the allergy-arthritis connection. To date, researchers have found no cause-and-effect connection between the two.[3] So how come some people with arthritis report improvement in joint pain when they eliminate certain foods from their diets? The answer is that allergens suppress the immune system, allowing bacteria to flourish and intensify, thus adversely affecting the joints. When allergens are removed from the diet, the immune system is relieved of this burden and is better able to keep infection under control. Consequently, inflammation and pain diminish.

The next question: If allergies are not directly involved, how does fasting improve joint pain? The answer is simple. Studies show that it is not the removal of supposed allergens during a fast that improves arthritic symptoms, but the fact that fasting tempers inflammation.[4] During a fast, inflammation is quieted down throughout the body, including in the joint tissues and even in infected teeth and gums.[5] Without the inflammation, the pain lessens or even goes away. When foods are again consumed, inflammation returns and so does the pain.

If allergies were the cause of arthritis, then an extended fast should completely clear up symptoms during the fast when the body is free from the antagonizing food. However, fasting does not usually result in a complete removal of symptoms. The pain may lessen significantly, but not completely go away. Therefore, allergy is not the culprit.

Allergies can depress your immune system and trigger or, rather, intensify the conditions that result in joint pain. Identifying and eliminating allergens from your diet may be helpful but is not a complete solution. Although allergies can play a role in aggravating arthritis, they do not cause it.

Joan had suffered with agonizing pain from rheumatoid arthritis in her hands and left knee for four years. Drugs she was taking to control her symptoms complicated her life by causing digestive disturbances. Then one day, she read an article regarding the connection between allergies and arthritis. Suspecting allergies were the cause of her problem, she began to phase out the arthritis drugs she was taking and to evaluate her diet. "I analyzed my eating habits," says Joan. "I strongly suspected I was reacting to bread, sugar, tomatoes, hamburger, and coffee. I went right ahead and just cut out those foods completely. I did feel slightly uncomfortable for a few days without my favorite foods. But after a week, the arthritis began to improve, quite noticeably. And for the first time in years, my digestive pains cleared up completely. I still had low level arthritis pain and stiffness. But I was really elated with my success." She consulted with a doctor who tested her for allergies and discovered she was allergic to wheat, sugar, beef, and coffee, but not tomato. Although some pain remains, Joan has recovered much of the mobility in her hands and knee. The removal of the allergens improved Joan's immune function, allowing her body to better defend itself against infection. The infection causing her arthritis, while calmed down, still holds on. Many people, like Joan, swear they had success with allergen elimination, but this is only a band-aid solution and the results are variable. Some patients show dramatic improvement, while others show little or none.

Researchers have found that, after a prolonged fast, if patients return to their normal eating habits, arthritis soon returns to the same level it was before the fast. If, however, they go on a vegetarian diet, rich in fresh fruits and vegetables and low in grains (gluten-free), arthritis symptoms remain suppressed for as long as 1-2 years.[6] The benefit is not due to the elimination of allergens, but is a result of keeping inflammation under control and of the elimination of certain troublesome foods, which we will talk about shortly.[7]

Many people find that eliminating "junk" foods from their diets brings about significant improvement, whether they are allergic to these foods or not. Marjorie, 62, suffered for 10 years with increasing pain in her hands from rheumatoid arthritis. The drugs she was given were of little help. Finally, her hands became so stiff and swollen that she underwent surgery. After the operation, Marjorie's fingers became even stiffer than they were before. She felt helpless. Drugs didn't work, surgery didn't work; there was little hope for her. By chance, she learned of natural therapies for arthritis treatment that focused on the diet and decided to give them a try. Marjorie visited a doctor who specialized in natural medicine. The doctor was appalled when she divulged all of the health-destroying foods she was eating. The doctor put her on a purification diet designed to detoxify her body. Six days after she stopped eating her usual foods, Marjorie was astounded to find herself completely free of pain. At this point, she was placed on a diet of fresh fruits and vegetables. Eight days later, she regained the full use of her hands. The doctor advised her to permanently adopt a dietary regimen of fresh, natural, high-fiber foods. Since then, Marjorie has stayed on the new diet and remains pain-free without experiencing any flare-ups. She leads an active normal life, uninhibited by joint pain, and loves eating healthfully. Unlike those who simply eliminate dietary allergens, Marjorie was completely freed from her crippling arthritis.

There are foods that promote poor health and arthritis and foods that promote good health and prevent arthritis. Which are which? When you ask someone what constitutes a "healthy" diet, you will get any number of answers ranging from vegetarian to low-carb to blood type and macrobiotic diets. The following section provides the clue to recognizing healthy and unhealthy diets.

Diseases of Modern Civilization

Arthritis, along with periodontal disease (gum disease), tooth decay (cavities), fibromyalgia, heart disease, diabetes, cancer, asthma, and many other common health problems are typically referred to as the "diseases of modern civilization." This term was coined to describe a phenomenon that has been identified by numerous doctors, anthropologists, and researchers over the past century. It has been observed that people in rural communities living and working as they have for hundreds or thousands of years rarely experience these health problems. However, when they come into contact with civilization and adopt modern ways or move to the cities, they begin to develop the same types of degenerative diseases found in these communities.

For instance, British surgeon Denis Burkitt, MD, spent nearly two decades working in rural Africa. Beginning in the 1940s, Burkitt observed that the health of the rural Africans was much better overall than that of the British or Europeans who also resided there. They lived in the same climate, but their eating habits were very different. The rural Africans ate traditional foods, while the British maintained their love of white bread, jams, jelly, tea, and such. Burkitt noticed that as native Africans adopted Western ways and foods (became more "civilized"), they started to develop the same diseases experienced by the Europeans.

In the South Pacific, Ian Prior, MD, studied the native Pacific Islanders in the 1960s and witnessed the exact same thing. As long as the islanders maintained their traditional native lifestyle and diet, they did not experience the diseases of modern civilization. Yet, when they migrated to New Zealand or Australia, they quickly acquired the same degenerative diseases of their adopted countries.

Anthropologist Vihjalmur Stefansson, working among the Eskimos of Northern Canada and Alaska from 1906-1918, witnessed the very same thing. When he first came among them, they had very little contact with "white men" and civilization and were completely free from "white man's" diseases. There was no arthritis, tooth decay,

100

diabetes, or cancer among them. When the Eskimo began living in villages and became exposed to modern foods, all of that changed.

This same phenomenon is seen in the archeological record as well. The skeletal remains of rural inhabitants throughout most of the world show few signs of modern degenerative diseases. However, as civilization develops, diseases of civilization begin to occur. It is interesting that wherever dental disease is evident, arthritis is present also. The diseases go hand-in-hand throughout history. Mummies of the royalty and the privileged class of Egypt often show signs of tooth decay and arthritis, even more so than those of the lower class who lived a more meager existence and probably had a lifestyle similar to rural dwellers.

It is apparent that diet plays a very important role in the development of poor health and arthritis. The diet you eat can cause arthritis or it can prevent it. Below, we'll look at the type of diet that promotes poor health. I call this the "Arthritis Forming Diet," because if you follow this course of eating, chances are high that you will eventually develop some form of arthritis.

The Arthritis Forming Diet

If you want to destroy your health and develop arthritis or fibromyalgia you should include in your meals and snacks the following items:

Pancakes and waffles
Syrup
Jellies and jams
Cold breakfast cereal
Toaster pastries
Donuts
White bread
Bagels
Muffins
Cinnamon rolls
Granola bars
Fruit juice (apple, orange, grape, etc.)
Pasta (spaghetti, lasagna, macaroni and cheese, etc.)
Pizza

101

Fries
Potato chips
Corn chips
Crackers
Processed meats (salami, bologna, hot dogs, chicken nuggets, etc.)
White rice
Frozen dinners
Canned foods
Restaurant foods
Cookies
Cake
Pie
Candy and chocolate
Soda
Coffee
Alcohol
Powdered fruit-flavored drinks (Tang, Kool-aid, etc.)
Sports drinks
Energy drinks
Sugar
Artificial sweeteners
Vegetable oils
Margarine
Vegetable shortening
Low-fat or fat-free dairy (milk, cheese, etc.)

Yikes! What a list. Are these the foods you normally eat every day? If they are, and you don't already have arthritis, you are an arthritis victim just waiting to happen. People are generally surprised when they look at this list of foods because it includes items most of us eat every day, seven days a week, week after week, year after year. In the long run you will suffer. Arthritis is one of the symptoms that may occur as your health declines.

Some of you may be wondering, if you eliminate all of the above foods, what else is there to eat?...Lots! Such as "real" foods like fresh fruits, vegetables, nuts, seeds, whole grains, whole dairy, eggs, and fresh unprocessed meats. Some may say, "Well, I already eat fruits and vegetables and eat whole grains whenever I can." However, those who say this are often overweight, too, as are some 60 percent of Americans. *If you are overweight, you are eating an arthritis forming diet!*

So what exactly constitutes a healthy diet? We can call it "The Anti-Arthritis Diet" as described below.

Better Health with the Anti-Arthritis Diet

The definition of a "healthy" way of eating is not a vegetarian diet or low-carb diet or any particular diet that happens to be currently in vogue. The key to really understanding what constitutes a healthy diet was discovered by Weston A. Price, DDS, back in the late 1930s. In his practice as a dentist he observed that later in his career, he was seeing more and more patients with dental and health problems that were rare when he first started practicing dentistry. Early in his career, people ate mostly foods fresh from local farms and ranches. As people began to leave the farms and move into the cities to find work, there came a demand for more food and better distribution and preservation. As a result, food technology began to change. Foods entered the era of mass production and were processed, canned, packaged, and otherwise prepared to have a long storage life so they would be easy to store and transport. In this process, the nutritional value of the foods declined and questionable ingredients were added. Our entire diet began to change dramatically from fresh to processed and packaged.

Dr. Price theorized that the decline in nutrition was the cause of this dramatic increase in disease, particularly degenerative diseases like arthritis, heart disease, and diabetes. To test his theory, he spent nearly a decade traveling around the world studying indigenous peoples, their diets, and how what they ate affected their health. He traveled to remote regions of Canada and Alaska, the Pacific Islands, Australia, Africa, South America, and isolated regions in Europe. When he went into an area he would examine the teeth of the people and note their general health and the types of diseases they had or didn't have. He also recorded the foods they ate and even analyze them for their nutritional content. He would locate people who were completely

103

isolated and uninfluenced by modern civilization. In the 1930s there were still many people who had not embraced modern civilization and continued to live their traditional ways and eat their traditional foods.

Dr. Price discovered that those people who ate their traditional foods had extraordinarily good dental health and excellent overall health. They did not suffer from arthritis, asthma, diabetes, heart disease, cancer, or any of the so-called diseases of modern civilization. However, when these very same people began to adopt Western ways and modern foods, their dental and overall health quickly declined. It didn't take much to cause a change. As traders visited these people they would acquire only a few items such as white flour, sugar, canned meat, and vegetable oils. Although these "modern" foods may have constituted only 10 or 20 percent of their entire diet, their health was significantly affected. The more they adopted Western foods, the greater the degree of their physical degeneration.

Dr. Price saw this pattern in *every* population he studied. There were no exceptions. The evidence was clear. People eating whole foods, as they had for thousands of years, were robust and healthy. When they began to replace their traditional foods with modern, processed foods, their health declined.

One of the things Dr. Price did when he evaluated the people's health was to carefully examine and document the conditions of their teeth and mouths. Cavities and gum disease were relatively rare among those eating traditional diets. These people *never* brushed their teeth, never used dental floss, nor did they use mouthwash, yet their teeth were in far better condition than any of those he saw in his practice in Ohio. He observed that when these people began to add a little sugar and white flour into their diets, their dental health quickly declined. Their mouths became ravaged with cavities and disease. They also started to develop arthritis and other degenerative conditions. *Diet*, Dr. Price discovered, *was the most important factor affecting a person's dental and physical health.* His findings were published in 1939 in a book titled *Nutrition and Physical Degeneration*.

Dr. Price studied populations with a wide variety of climates, cultures, customs, and dietary practices. The foods the people ate encompassed a broad spectrum. Some populations were nearly total carnivores, consuming almost nothing but meat. Others relied almost entirely on dairy, and still others based their diets around whole grains or fruits. None of the diets, however, were vegetarian; all included meat or animal products of some type. There was nothing common among these indigenous groups except for the fact that the food was all fresh or minimally processed using traditional techniques, such as natural fermentation or drying. It didn't matter if the diet was mostly meat or grains or vegetables as long as the food was fresh and natural.

Sugar and Refined Grains

The two foods that Dr. Price found to have the greatest deleterious impact on health were sugar and white flour. Today science has clearly shown that sugar is public enemy number one when it comes to cavities and gum disease. We are cautioned not to eat too much, or it will rot our teeth. This is true, but few people really pay any attention. They go on and eat sugar without a second thought. In 1800 sugar consumption consisted of about 10 pounds per person a year.[8] Today each person consumes on average of about 160 pounds a year. That's almost half a pound of sugar a day—and our teeth show it! Approximately 98 percent of the population has some level of tooth decay or gum disease. Even regular brushing and flossing hasn't reversed the destruction caused by sugar.

Refined sugar isn't the only culprit. White flour is just as bad. White flour is made primarily of starch. Starch is composed entirely of sugar. The only difference is that in starch, the sugar molecules are all linked together in a chain but, once we eat it, our digestive enzymes break the links into individual sugar molecules. So, eating a slice of white bread is essentially the equivalent of eating a couple of spoonfuls of sugar. White bread begins to turn into sugar in our mouths as we chew it. Saliva contains digestive enzymes that immediately begin to transform the starch into sugar.

Sugar, whether in pure form or as white flour, feeds oral bacteria. The bacteria in our mouths absolutely love sugar. The more sugar you eat, the more they eat, and consequently, the faster they grow and multiply, and the sooner they can overrun the mouth causing infection and disease. As long as you eat sugar and white flour (and other refined grains), you are feeding disease-causing bacteria in your mouth. Sugar is like a fertilizer for bacteria. The more you stuff into your mouth, the heartier they grow.

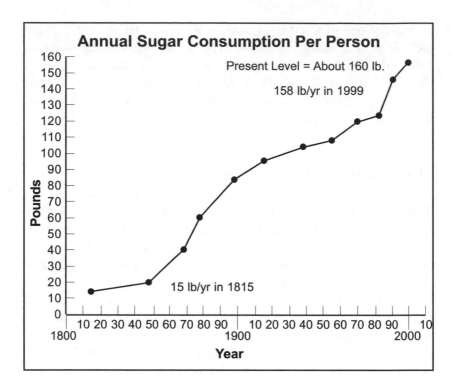

Annual Sugar Consumption Per Person

Present Level = About 160 lb.

158 lb/yr in 1999

15 lb/yr in 1815

Pounds

Year

The people whom Dr. Price studied, who ate traditional diets, consumed few, if any, sweets. Their teeth were in excellent shape even without the benefit of any dental hygiene or dentists. Their teeth were healthy because they ate right.

Traditional Fats and Processed Vegetable Oils

Another modern food that wreaked havoc on people's health was processed vegetable oil. Animal fats and butter were the most commonly used oils in these societies and had been used for generations with no detrimental effects. Next in importance were olive, coconut, and palm oils. All of these were relatively easy to extract using primitive methods. Vegetable oils from seeds, such as soybean and safflower oils, were much more difficult to extract and process and, therefore, were rarely used until after the invention of the hydraulic press in the late 1800s. Processed vegetable oils were seldom used

106

until the twentieth century. With the invention of the hydrogenation process in 1901, liquid vegetable oils were transformed into solid fats. These fats were sold as margarine and shortening and promoted as cheaper alternatives to animal fats.

We hear a lot about how good polyunsaturated vegetable oils are for us. What consumers don't know is that these vegetable oils are far more harmful than saturated fats. Over the past two decades, mountains of research have confirmed this. Researchers have found that the consumption of polyunsaturated vegetable oil constituting only 10 percent of total calories can lead to blood disorders, cancer, liver damage, and vitamin deficiencies. Excessive consumption has been linked to:

- Lowered resistance to infectious disease by depressing the immune system, killing white blood cells, which defend us against harmful microorganisms and cancerous cells.

- Higher risk for heart disease because they increase inflammation, elevate blood pressure, and encourage blood clotting.

- Increased incidence of asthma, eczema, and allergic rhinitis, which mirrors the decline in use of saturated fats and the corresponding switch to polyunsaturated fats.

- Impaired brain functions such as learning ability, memory, cognitive functions, and behaviour, possibly leading to Alzheimer's disease, Parkinson's disease, senile dementia, dyslexia and perhaps even attention deficit disorder.

- Skyrocketing incidence of blindness due to age-related macular degeneration in the United States, Canada, Australia, and most other industrialized countries.

- Development of allergies, psoriasis, defective blood glucose regulation, migraine headaches, and autoimmune and inflammatory conditions including rheumatoid arthritis, irritable bowel syndrome, multiple sclerosis, lupus nephritis, and certain inflammatory kidney conditions.

Polyunsaturated fats are highly vulnerable to oxidation. When exposed to heat, light, or oxygen, they spontaneously oxidize and form destructive molecules known as free radicals. These free radicals are highly reactive and attack unsaturated fats and proteins. In turn, these substances become oxidized and generate more free radicals. It is a self-perpetuating process.

When oil is extracted from seeds, the oxidation process is set in motion and continues right through to bottling and even during distribution. When used in cooking, oxidation and the formation of destructive free radicals are greatly accelerated.

Oxidation occurs inside the body as well. Our only defense against free radicals is antioxidants. Fresh foods contain antioxidant nutrients such as vitamins A, C, and E, beta-carotene, and the minerals zinc and selenium.

In contrast, saturated fats are very resistant to oxidation. They act more like protective antioxidants because they prevent oxidation and the formation of free radicals.

Monounsaturated fatty acids are more stable than polyunsaturated fatty acids but less stable than saturated fatty acids. Replacing polyunsaturated fats with saturated and monounsaturated fats can help reduce the risks associated with free radicals. Eating a diet rich in antioxidant nutrients can help against the oxidation of polyunsaturated fatty acids in the body.

Most cooks recommend polyunsaturated vegetable oils in cooking and food preparation as a "healthy" alternative to butter, coconut oil, or other saturated fats.

Ironically, these unsaturated vegetable oils, when used in cooking, form a variety of toxic compounds that are far more damaging to health than any saturated fat could ever be. As it turns out, polyunsaturated vegetable oils are the least suitable for cooking.

Any unsaturated vegetable oil can become toxic when heated. And even a small amount, especially if eaten frequently over time, will affect health. Oxidized oils have been found to induce damage to interstitial tissues and blood vessel walls and to cause numerous organ lesions in animals. Researchers are now beginning to recognize that heated vegetable oils are far more harmful to the heart and circulatory system than excess cholesterol or animal fats.

Vegetable oil consumption has a direct impact on arthritis. These oils depress the immune system, thus increasing the risk of infection or reducing the ability to fight chronic infection. They also promote inflammation, thus aggravating arthritic conditions. Too much polyunsaturated vegetable oils in the diet is known to adversely affect arthritic knee joints.[9]

Even more detrimental to health than processed vegetable oils are the hydrogenated vegetable oils—margarine and shortening. During the process of hydrogenation, artificial fats known as *trans fatty acids* are created. These are some of the worst fats you can eat. Trans fatty acids are now known to contribute to heart disease, diabetes, stroke, cancer, autoimmune disease, and a host of other health problems. Stay away from them. Hydrogenated or partially hydrogenated oils are often used in food processing. Read ingredient labels and avoid all foods that contain them.

Over the past several decades, we have been advised to avoid fats and oils that contain high amounts of saturated fat because saturated fats increase blood cholesterol levels. When the cholesterol theory of heart disease was proposed in the 1960s, it was believed that cholesterol in the blood accumulated and clogged arteries, which in turn led to heart attacks. Since that time, the cholesterol theory of heart disease has proven to be untrue. The plaque that forms in arteries consists of protein, blood platelets, calcium, and cholesterol. The main component is protein, not cholesterol. Cholesterol is present because the body uses it to repair damage in the artery wall. It doesn't cause the clogging or the damage, it is there as a means to facilitate healing. It is guilty only by association.

High cholesterol is considered a marker or *risk factor* for heart disease, but not the cause. There are many risk factors for heart disease; a lack of exercise and being male are two other risk factors. But like cholesterol, neither a lack of exercise nor being male causes heart disease. Risk factors simply indicate an increased risk of developing heart disease. The more risk factors you have, the greater your risk or your chance of suffering a heart attack. There are a dozen or so known risk factors for heart disease. High cholesterol is only one of them, and it isn't even the strongest or most important. Half of all those people who suffer heart attacks have normal to below normal blood cholesterol levels. So, obviously high cholesterol does not cause the attacks. We hear a lot about cholesterol these days because drug companies make billions of dollars a year selling cholesterol-lowering drugs. Consequently, they spend millions of dollars each year promoting the need to lower cholesterol. Drug makers admit that simply lowering cholesterol does not lower the incidence of heart attacks. Read the fine print in the advertising, that is one of the statements that is often included.

People around the world eating traditional diets have relied heavily on foods rich in cholesterol and saturated fat. These people never had heart disease, high blood pressure, or strokes until they replaced their traditional fats for processed vegetable oils and other modern foods.

Diet Summary

To sum up what we learn from Dr. Price's work, the best foods for achieving and maintaining good dental and overall health are fresh fruits, vegetables, nuts, seeds, eggs, whole grains, whole dairy, unprocessed meats, and healthy traditional oils. Traditional oils include olive, coconut, and palm oils along with animal fats and butter. Foods should be eaten raw and cooked, and be of both vegetable and animal origin.

Sugar is one of the most health damaging foods and the so-called "natural" sugars aren't much better. Sugar includes white table sugar (sucrose), brown sugar, honey, molasses, maple syrup, corn syrup, Sucanat, date sugar, glucose, fructose, and high fructose corn syrup, and anything that is used as a sweetening agent.

White flour is not much different from sugar. White flour includes any and all refined grains and the products made with them including bread, cookies, crackers, pastries, rolls, muffins, etc.

Refined vegetable oils include almost all of the oils sold in the grocery store including corn, soybean, canola, safflower, sunflower, peanut, and cottonseed oils and margarine and vegetable shortening as well as hydrogenated and partially hydrogenated oils.

The more processing a food undergoes, the more nutrients are lost and the more likely that unhealthy ingredients have been added. Chemical additives are not foods but foreign substances, toxins that the body has to process and eliminate. Processed foods deprive the body of good nutrition and depress immune function, making you more vulnerable to infection and poor health. If a food is cooked and is sold in a can, plastic, box, foil, or other sealed wrapping, it likely isn't fit to eat. If a product has more than four or five ingredients, or if the ingredients consist of multisyllabic words you can't pronounce, like butylated hydroxytoluene, then it's best to leave it alone.

Changing your present diet to a more natural, traditional one can be one of the most effective steps you can take in overcoming arthritis. Cutting out sugar and white flour will starve the troublesome bacteria in your mouth, hitting the problem squarely between the eyes.

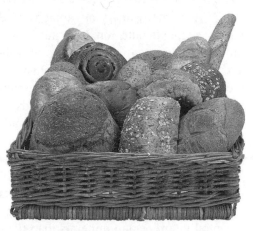

After suffering for three years with increasing pain from rheumatoid arthritis, 41-year-old E. C.'s knees became so crippled she had to give up her job as a teacher and take to a wheelchair. She tried all the usual drugs without success. Frustrated with the poor results from her doctors, E. C. went to a natural practitioner. He put her on a seven-day fast followed by a diet of fresh, whole foods. By the end of the last day of the fast her arthritis pains had gone away. Two weeks later, after following a whole foods diet program, almost all of the swelling had also disappeared. Exactly six weeks after her first visit with the natural health practitioner, E. C. was able to stand up out of her wheelchair and walk—entirely free of stiffness and pain. Three months later she was back at school teaching.

Eating a healthy diet can have a very pronounced effect in both preventing and reversing arthritis. For most people, eating a whole foods diet is totally new to them and challenging. The first step is to understand what constitutes a whole food. Once you understand that,

111

then you can focus on creating delicious, satisfying meals based around these foods. Although the concept of whole foods is simple, many people don't fully understand it. For this reason, I have included a whole foods learning challenge to help teach you how to eat healthfully. The challenge describes whole foods in more detail and includes a seven-day hands-on trial, with an evaluation afterward. The details are found in the Appendix.

Good Nutrition Fights Arthritis

One of the primary advantages of eating a whole foods diet is getting adequate nutrition. Poor nutrition can have a significant impact on the development and progress of arthritis as well as gum disease and many other health problems. Just because you may eat three full meals a day and may even be overweight doesn't mean you are well nourished. Because most of the foods we eat are vitamin deficient, we can eat and eat and even overeat and still be malnourished. Most North Americans do not get the recommended daily dose of all of the essential vitamins and minerals. We eat a lot of food, but we don't get the nutrients we need. Some of the foods we eat, such as sugar and vegetable oils, actually drain nutrients from our bodies.

Studies show that arthritis sufferers have lower levels of many essential vitamins and minerals than the general population, strongly suggesting that they do not eat properly. For example, in a study of gout patients, it was discovered that they had greater blood levels of homocysteine than normal, indicating deficiencies in B vitamins, particularly folic acid, B-12, and B-6.[10]

In another study, the effect of niacinamide, one of the B vitamins, was tested on osteoarthritis patients. Researchers found that supplementation with this vitamin resulted in a significant reduction in inflammation and improvement in joint flexibility,[11] thus indicating a deficiency in this important nutrient.

Vitamins C, E, B-1, B-2, B-6, and B-12 have shown to exert an inhibiting effect on osteoarthritis, again indicating a deficiency of these vitamins in the diet.[12]

A lack of vitamins D and K and the minerals calcium, magnesium, boron, zinc, and selenium can weaken bone and joint tissue, increasing

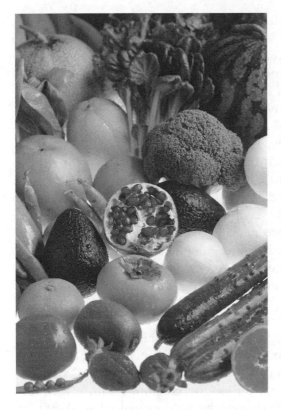

risk of osteoarthritis. For example, in geographic areas where boron intakes are low, arthritis incidence is high, and vice versa. Also, some studies have shown that boron supplementation can have a beneficial effect on osteoarthritis.[13]

Studies indicate that individuals with rheumatoid arthritis have low levels of vitamin C in their bodies.[14] A lack of adequate vitamin C hinders immune function. It also indicates that the immune system is under stress, probably because it is fighting a chronic infection. Vitamin C is also essential in forming collagen, which is needed to build and repair bone and joint tissues. Eating vitamin C-rich foods and even taking dietary supplements supplying 500 mg or more of vitamin C could be helpful.

Research shows that eating whole foods enhances the efficiency of the immune system. Rheumatoid arthritis patients often have chronic or repeated subclinical urinary tract infections. This can be seen by the presence of *Proteus mirabilis* bacteria in the urine. When rheumatoid arthritis patients are placed on a whole foods diet and symptoms improve, bacteria count in the urine also declines.[15]

You also need to eat an adequate amount of good fat every day. We currently live in an anti-fat society. Everyone seems to be afraid of eating fat in fear that it will make them fat or give them heart disease. Well, if the primary source of fat in your diet is processed vegetable oils and hydrogenated fats, then yes, this is true. But traditional fats promote health and are even essential for achieving proper nutrition.

Fat is an essential component of our bodies and is found in all our tissues. Our brains consist of 60 percent fat and cholesterol. All of your cells are encased in fatty membranes. Fat is used to produce energy and as a building block for tissues. Studies show that the body can convert fat (saturated and monounsaturated fats) into cartilage.[16] So, fat may be useful in keeping your joints healthy and limber.

An adequate amount of dietary fat is necessary for proper digestion and nutrient absorption. Fats delay the movement of food through the stomach and digestive system. This allows more time for foods to bathe in stomach acids and stay in contact with digestive enzymes. As a consequence, more nutrients, especially minerals which are normally tightly bound to other compounds, are released from our foods and absorbed into the body. Low-fat diets are actually detrimental because they prevent complete digestion of food and limit nutrient absorption.

Low-fat diets can promote mineral deficiencies. Calcium, for example, needs fat for proper absorption. For this reason, low-fat diets encourage osteoporosis and osteoarthritis. It is interesting that we often eat low-fat foods, including non-fat and low-fat milk, to get calcium; yet, by eating reduced fat milks, the calcium is not effectively absorbed. This may be one reason why people can drink loads of low-fat milk and take calcium supplements but still suffer from osteoporosis.

Fat is also required for the absorption of fat-soluble vitamins. These include Vitamins A, D, E, and K, and important phytonutrients and antioxidants such as beta-carotene. Too little fat in the diet can lead to serious nutritional deficiencies.

In most countries, fat consumption ranges from 20-40 percent of total calories. Health experts often recommend limiting fat calories to 30 percent or less because of their belief in the outdated cholesterol theory and fear of heart disease. However, studies on populations that exceed this limit do not show any higher incidence of heart disease than those who eat less total fat.[17]

Obesity is often associated with osteoarthritis. People who are overweight eat the wrong kinds of foods. Many overweight people

114

don't necessarily overeat, but what they do eat builds body fat. Natural foods are not fattening. They are filling and satisfying, so overeating is not a problem.

Taking a vitamin and mineral supplement may or may not be helpful. Many people rely on dietary supplements to supply them with the nutrients they need. Consequently, they feel less inclined to eat well, thinking the supplement will make up for a poor diet. This is not the case. Dietary supplements are just that—supplements. They are not foods. They are taken to supplement an otherwise adequate diet, not make up for it.

Many studies have been reported recently that dietary supplements aren't as protective against degenerative diseases as they were once believed to be. Several studies have shown no particular benefit in taking vitamins for the prevention of certain diseases like heart disease or cancer. We still need the vitamins and minerals, but supplements are not the best way to get them. Studies do, however, consistently show that getting your vitamins and minerals from eating whole foods does protect against a myriad of diseases. So, it is to your favor that you don't rely on supplements, but get your nutrition from foods—real foods.

Low-Carb Whole Foods Diet

Your first step in making wise dietary choices is to transition to a whole foods diet. If eating this way is new to you, take the Seven-Day Whole Foods Challenge described in the Appendix. This is a good learning tool and will show you how well you understand the whole foods concept. It could also be an eye-opener for you and reveal just how much processed food you really eat.

If you have active tooth decay or gum disease and joint or muscle pain, you might benefit even more quickly by going a step further by adopting a low-carb whole foods diet. While the whole foods diet is one that you should adopt for life, the low-carb whole foods diet is a therapy. It, too, can be practiced for life, but need not be. The benefit of the low-carb diet is that it eliminates from the diet foods that are most likely to promote oral infections.

115

During his worldwide study, Dr. Price found that those indigenous people who had the best dental health were those who ate low-carb diets. The Eskimos, for instance, whose diet consisted almost entirely of meat and fish (extremely low-carb) had the least number of cavities of all the groups he studied. Those who ate primarily grains, even whole grains, and a little honey, had the most cavities. Although their teeth were by far better than any group that ate modern foods, among the indigenous groups, they had the least resistance to decay.

Since good dental health is imperative to conquering arthritis and fibromyalgia, you might consider taking the whole foods concept a step further and go into the low-carb realm. Low-carbing requires more will-power because there are more restrictions on what you can and cannot eat. However, your fight against arthritis will be better fought and you will have quicker results.

In a low-carb whole foods diet, consumption of carbohydrate-rich foods is strictly limited. The high-carb foods include all grains, all natural sweeteners, starchy vegetables, and to some extent sweet fruits and dairy. Grains include wheat, rice, corn, barley, oats, etc. Natural sweeteners include honey, molasses, dehydrated sugarcane juice, date sugar, etc. Starchy vegetables include potatoes, sweet potatoes, winter squash, beans, and peas. In a true low-carb diet, all of these foods would be entirely eliminated.

The primary foods you would eat include meat, fish, eggs, good fats and oils, and vegetables—lots of fresh raw and cooked vegetables; raw salads, steamed, and stir-fried vegetables. Vegetables prepared and cooked in all types of ways and seasoned with herbs, spices, fats and butter, cheeses, and meat juices. Hard and soft cheeses are okay, so is cream, but milk, even whole milk, has a fair amount of sugar (lactose) and should be limited. Unsweetened yogurt is okay, but not sweetened. The low-carb diet is supplemented with small amounts of nuts, seeds, and low-sugar fruits (berries). Herbs and spices, herbal teas, water with lemon, and unsweetened condiments (vinegar, mustard, pickles, etc.) are also permitted.

After you start low-carbing, don't be surprised if you begin to lose excess weight. This is one of the pleasant side effects to the whole foods low-carb diet. Since you eliminate foods that promote weight gain and eat more nutrient-dense foods that satisfy hunger, you tend to eat less and consume fewer calories. Consequently, excess body fat begins to melt off. In a few months, you could lose 10, 20, or more pounds, depending on how much excess weight you began with. Losing excess pounds is definitely a step toward better health and relieves stress on your body. Your aching joints will thank you.

Once your health starts to improve and your joint and muscle pain diminish, you can add back into your diet whole grains, natural sweeteners, starchy vegetables, fruits, and milk. But if you want to keep your joints healthy, you need to maintain good eating habits. Bad habits are what caused your problems in the first place. If you go back to your same old eating habits, it won't be long until you end up in trouble again. It is like hitting your hand with a hammer. When you stop hitting yourself, the pain will go away and your hand will heal. If you start hitting your hand again, you are going to feel it. The pain is going to return. You can't eat an arthritis forming diet and expect to avoid arthritis or fibromyalgia.

"After following your program for several weeks I was overjoyed to see the pain in my toes vanish," says Ian R. "When Christmas season came around a couple of months later I let up on my healthy diet a bit and indulged in the holiday treats. I received a couple of boxes of chocolates and various other goodies that I just couldn't pass up. For about three weeks I ate more sweets than I probably had all year. When January rolled around I noticed something disturbing happen, the pain in my toes began to return. It persisted for several weeks. At first I didn't know why this was happening, but then I realized what I had been eating prior to the relapse. I immediately removed all sweets and grains from my diet and increased my meat, fat, and coconut oil consumption. Within a few weeks the pain went away."

An excellent resource for preparing and cooking whole foods and even low-carb whole foods is the book *Nourishing Traditions* by Sally Fallon and Mary Enig. Another good book is *Real Food: What to Eat and Why* by Nina Planck.

Chapter 8

Rebuilding Damaged Joints

Edna, a 62-year old church volunteer, was getting into her car after work one evening when she felt a slight pain in her hip. She paid little attention to it. A week later however, the pain became noticeably more intense and occurred with more frequency. Before long, it felt "like someone was hitting me there with a hammer!" she said. "Just getting out of the chair to go to the bathroom was torture." She stopped her daily walks and the gardening she used to enjoy.

The doctor diagnosed her with osteoarthritis. He told her that there wasn't much he could do except to help relieve some of the symptoms, but she was going to have to deal with this for the rest of her life. He gave her various medications to calm the symptoms. Side effects of the drugs, however, caused her to develop frequent headaches, blurred her vision, and eventually damaged her liver. Despite the treatment, the pain in her hip still persisted. "Life used to be fun," she said. "Now it's hell."

Edna heard about a dietary supplement called glucosamine/ chondroitin that was reported to help those suffering from arthritis. She figured she didn't have anything to lose; it was not a drug and surely wouldn't have the deleterious side effects she was experiencing with the prescribed medications. She purchased the supplement from her local grocery and began taking it daily.

After the first week she hadn't noticed any improvement in her symptoms. She began to think that it wasn't going to work and decided to stop taking it at the end of day nine. But when she woke up on day 10 her hip felt a little better, so she kept taking it. On day 15 she reported that her hip felt 25 percent better and on day 20 it felt 50 percent better. After a few more weeks, she was able to resume her daily walks and work in her garden again. She discontinued her medications and no longer has to deal with their troubling side effects.

Edna, like many other arthritis sufferers, discovered the miracle of glucosamine and chondroitin. Over the past couple of decades a substantial number of studies have been published describing the effectiveness of glucosamine/chondroitin in treating arthritis, and in particular osteoarthritis. As part of your arthritis recovery program, glucosamine/chondroitin can be of tremendous benefit in rebuilding and speeding the healing of damaged joints.

The first step in beating arthritis is to stop the source of the infection. In most cases that source will be in your mouth. Once you have resolved your dental issues, bacteria no longer stream into your blood and attack joint tissue. This allows your body's own recuperative powers to take over and fight off the remaining infection in your body and rebuild damaged joint tissue. Joints damaged by years of degeneration, if not completely destroyed, will heal.

Eating a healthy diet, keeping the teeth and mouth clean and disease free, and supporting a healthy immune system will aid your body in rebuilding and healing damaged joints. If your joints have undergone extensive damage, you can enhance your body's reconstructive efforts and speed the healing by feeding it the basic building blocks necessary to reconstruct the joint tissues.

Let's look at the analogy of building a house with rebuilding arthritic joints. If you build a house you will need lumber, nails, bricks, carpet, and other materials. If the building supply company delivers only half of the bricks that you need, you can't complete the construction, no matter how many extra nails or rolls of carpet he brings. You need a precise amount of each building material, and the material must be in a form you can use. If the supply company brings a load of two-foot-long boards and you need them to be 10 feet long, the job still can't be completed, even though the boards are made of the right material. So the form of the materials you receive must be correct as well.

Our diet supplies our bodies with the building blocks it needs to build and repair tissues. If the diet lacks certain nutritional building blocks, then the work remains incomplete. And the longer the repair job remains unfinished, the greater the risk of further damage. As more damage occurs, there is a need for even more building blocks.

Years ago doctors discovered that eating organ meats had a therapeutic effect on certain health problems. This led to the concept of "like heals like." In other words, if a person had liver troubles, then eating calf liver or chicken liver could bring about healing. Likewise, if a person had heart or pancreas problems, the patient would be encouraged to eat heart or pancreas meats. Today, research now supports this concept.

The dietary supplement glucosamine/chondroitin follows this philosophy. Glucosamine and chondroitin are two basic building blocks found in the connective tissues of the joints. When consumed, they supply the exact type of materials our bodies need to repair the damage in arthritic joints. You can also get these building blocks simply by eating the cartilage that often accompanies meats. Cartilage is attached to the ends of joints. The white, rubber-like material on the ends of chicken bones, for example, is cartilage, just like that in your joints.

Many studies have shown that both glucosamine and chondroitin can significantly reduce pain and improve joint function in those with arthritis.[1-4] For example, one study looked at 80 patients all diagnosed with severe osteoarthritis.[5] During the 30-day, double-blind study, the participants were given either 1,500 milligrams of glucosamine or a placebo. Every week the researchers took measurements of the patients' pain, joint tenderness, swelling, and range of movement. They found that 73 percent of those taking the supplement experienced a significant reduction in overall symptoms. Within three weeks, the symptoms in the treatment group had declined by half. At the end of the trial, 20 percent reported complete relief from all symptoms. This study is typical of many that have been reported over the years.

Numerous double-blind studies have shown glucosamine and chondroitin to yield results as good as or even better than nonsteroidal anti-inflammatory drugs (NSAIDs) in relieving the pain and inflammation of osteoarthritis.[6-9]

Drugs relieve pain by blocking the signals the nerves send to the brain. The pain and the damage is still there; it is just not picked up by the brain. Neither glucosamine nor chondroitin have pain-relieving effects like drugs do. Research demonstrates that glucosamine and chondroitin are selectively taken up by joint tissue in rebuilding the joint. They work to reduce pain by repairing the damaged cartilage, thus reducing the irritation that causes inflammation and pain. In a study conducted in France, 50 patients suffering from osteoarthritis of the knee were given either chondroitin sulfate or pain medication. Cartilage tissue samples were taken at the beginning of the study and again after three months of therapy. The cartilage from the subjects taking the pain medication showed no improvement. However, those taking the chondroitin supplements showed that a significant degree of repair had taken place over the study period.[10]

The beneficial effects of glucosamine and chondroitin increase over time. Since the glucosamine and chondroitin do not actually block pain as drugs do, their effects on pain relief occur more slowly. Over time, however, their results can be greater and much longer lasting. For example, in one study the pain relieving effects of glucosamine were compared to ibuprofen.[11] Subjects taking ibuprofen reported an immediate reduction of pain. The level of pain relief quickly leveled off to about half of what it was at the beginning of the study. In the glucosamine group, pain gradually declined for the first two weeks and then more rapidly diminished thereafter, equaling the effects of ibuprofen after the third week and then showing a greater reduction of pain thereafter (see graph on next page). The results showed significantly better pain reduction with glucosamine than with ibuprofen. Other studies have shown very similar results, with pain being reduced by half after about three weeks.

Both glucosamine and chondroitin have been shown to effectively rebuild joint tissue and reduce pain, swelling, and inflammation caused by degenerative joint disease, especially osteoarthritis. However, when the two are used in combination, the effects are better than either one alone. They work synergistically together, each enhancing the healing effects of the other.

While pain medication and anti-inflammatory drugs are accompanied by serious side effects that may cause further damage,

121

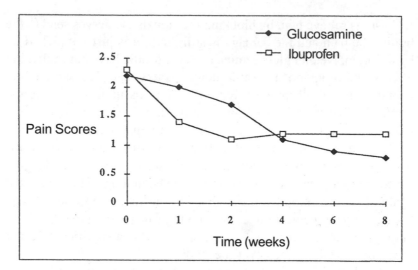

Comparison of pain relief between glucosamine and ibuprofen. At first ibuprofin is more effective at reducing pain. After three weeks glucosamine becomes more effective.

glucosamine and chondroitin have no harmful side effects and are completely safe.[12] After all, they are not drugs, but essentially just food.

You can get glucosamine/chondroitin in health food stores and pharmacies. You will find glucosamine and chondroitin in different forms such as glucosamine sulfate, glucosamine hydrochloride, glucosamine hydroiodide, etc. Look for a single supplement containing a combination supplying 1,500 mg of glucosamine *sulfate* and 1,200 mg of chondroitin *sulfate* per serving. You would take one serving daily. A serving may consist of two or three capsules. This dosage covers all those people who weigh between 120 and 200 pounds (54 and 90 kg). If you weigh less than 120 pounds (54 kg) you can take a little less, if you like. If you are over 200 pounds (90 kg) you can take a little more. Keep in mind that glucosamine and chondroitin are food components, not drugs, so there is no risk in overdosing. You can take three, four, five times the recommended amount without experiencing any side effects or being in any danger. Currently, there is no known level at which they would become toxic. That does not necessarily mean that more is better. Stick to the recommended dose given above unless advised differently by your doctor.

Although numerous studies have shown positive effects with glucosamine/chondroitin, some studies have been less than impressive. Discrepancies in these studies have been attributed primarily to the quality of the supplements used. Studies have revealed that a number of brands claiming to contain certain doses of glucosamine or chondroitin sulfate have significantly less than is claimed, or even none at all.[13] The most likely brands to err in label accuracy are those from small, little known companies. Therefore, you should stick with respected name brands that are known and trusted.

Vitamin C and the mineral manganese increase the effectiveness of both glucosamine and chondroitin and are also needed for good joint health. So choose a brand that also includes these nutrients or consider adding a multivitamin and mineral supplement to your daily routine.

You also get a small amount of glucosamine and chondroitin in your diet. They are found in most animal tissues, especially the cartilage or "gristle" around joints. When you cook a roast or a whole chicken in the oven and put the leftovers with the drippings into the refrigerator, the drippings turn into jelly-like substance. This is full of congealed connective tissue. It is essentially meat-flavored gelatin. This is basically the same as the Knox gelatin you buy in the store, but without the sugar and flavoring. In fact, unflavored gelatin is often sold as a dietary supplement for maintaining joint health. Some doctors recommend taking one to two ¼-ounce packets (about 2½ teaspoons per packet) a day for this purpose. You need not make "Jell-O" to eat the gelatin. You could, but usually that involves adding sugar or some other sweetener. All you need to do is simply add the gelatin to other foods such as beverages, soups, casseroles, gravies, eggs, homemade breads and other baked goods, etc. An easy way to take it is by mixing it in a little juice, water, milk, or broth.

Although many people have experienced remarkable improvement just by using glucosamine/chondroitin or gelatin, keep in mind that gelatin itself is not a cure. As long as the primary cause of the arthritis (infection) is not addressed, dietary supplementation will only bring temporary relief. Without solving the underlying problem, there is no guarantee that the condition will not return. You must remove the underlying infection if you want a real cure. However, after the infection has been removed, supplementation can be of enormous benefit in aiding the body in rebuilding damaged joints.

Chapter 9

The Magic of Motion

Move Arthritis Out of Your Life

People with arthritis are, in general, more sedentary than those without the disease. Part of the reason may be due to joint discomfort that discourages physical activity, but inactive people are more likely to develop arthritis.[1]

Motion is like adding lotion to your joints. Contrary to popular belief, movement and exercise are beneficial to arthritic joints. It was once believed that arthritis, particularly osteoarthritis, was a consequence of overuse, too much stress, or excessive exercise on the joints. This mistaken idea is still widely purported today. Look up any definition or description of osteoarthritis, and you will see it described as being caused by aging, wear and tear, or excessive physical stress. Although former joint injuries can promote osteoarthritis, overuse or age does not cause it. "Wear and tear" is just another name for "exercise," and exercise does not cause osteoarthritis.

Reasonable exercise, carried out within the limits of comfort, putting joints through normal motions, even over many years, need not lead to osteoarthritis. Many studies have now shown no significant association between moderate-to-intense physical activity and osteoarthritis in the general population.[2] In fact, just the opposite has been found. Physical activity helps to protect against arthritis. Even if arthritis is present, exercise strengthens arthritic joints, improves range of motion, and eases pain and inflammation.[3] Among older adults with knee osteoarthritis, engaging in moderate physical activity at least three times per week can reduce the risk of arthritis-related disability by 47 percent.[4]

Exercise provides many benefits including increased longevity, decreased risk of cardiovascular disease, improved psychological well-being, weight control and management, and greater fitness. It is also a therapy for the knees. It strengthens the front and back muscles (quadriceps and hamstrings, respectively) of the thighs and can help prevent knee trouble—especially in women, who are five to seven times more likely to suffer a torn anterior cruciate ligament (ACL), which is among the most serious knee problems.

The consensus among most doctors is that exercise is necessary for patients with *all* forms of arthritis.[5] Exercise is essential for good joint health. The bones, cartilage, tendons, and other tissues in the joints react to exercise and weight bearing by growing stronger and healthier. The body absorbs more calcium, deposits it in the bones, and creates thicker and sturdier support structures. Exercise builds muscles and increases muscle tone. This creates support across the joints and helps to stabilize them. The tendons as well as the ligaments gain strength when they are used.

Rest does just the opposite of exercise. It causes atrophy. It increases calcium loss from the bone, allows the muscles and tendons to weaken, fails to circulate nutrients and remove waste from cartilage, and accelerates joint degeneration. It also has a psychological disadvantage of encouraging dependency. Inactivity increases the risk of developing arthritis. Even a few weeks wearing a plaster cast may result in cartilage degeneration.

The cartilage inside the joint does not have a blood supply. It receives its oxygen and nourishment and gets rid of waste products by the action of compression and expansion resulting from physical activity. Fluid is squeezed into and out of the joint space through movement. The health of your cartilage depends on *motion* because without motion there is no nourishment delivered to the cartilage.

This is one of the major reasons why infection so frequently attacks joints. There is no blood supply to the joints, so circulation is limited. Inactivity encourages bacteria or viruses to collect with little interference from the immune system or from antibiotics circulating in the bloodstream.

The joints can be viewed somewhat like a large sponge. A sponge sitting untouched in a pan of water can remain stagnant, the water inside the sponge remaining where it is and the surrounding water remaining outside the sponge. Only when the sponge is squeezed to force the water out and then released to suck new water inside is there any exchange between the fluid inside the sponge and the surrounding liquid. Exercise is the process of squeezing the sponge. The more you exercise, the more fluid flows in and out of the sponge. Bacteria can collect inside the sponge and feel right at home regardless of what's happening around it. Even if disinfecting soaps or detergents are added to the pan of water, if the sponge is not squeezed, the detergent cannot effectively penetrate inside the sponge to kill the bacteria. Exercise is essential to facilitate the exchange of fluids. Likewise with our joints, exercise is essential to circulate oxygen, nutrients, antibodies, and antibiotics and to remove metabolic waste, toxins, and bacteria.

If your body is exposed to an influx of microorganisms that circulate in the bloodstream, one of the most likely spots for them to accumulate is the joints. If they are allowed to establish a homestead, protected from the harsh environment of the bloodstream, they will flourish. They and the toxins they produce eat away at the joint tissue, causing chronic inflammation, pain, swelling, and degeneration. Getting adequate exercise is essential in flushing the infection out of your joints.

Types of Exercise

What types of exercise should you do? Most forms of exercise that allow you to move your joints are of benefit as long as they do not cause pain or injury. Using sports as your primary mode of exercise is not recommended because they are often too intense and are apt to cause injury. Avoid high-tension exercises that exert excessive force to the joints, such as weight lifting or running. Low-impact aerobic type exercises are the best. Weight-bearing exercises that utilize your body's weight are helpful in strengthing joint tissues in the ankles, knees, and hips.

If a movement is painful, don't do it. Exercise to the full range of motion of the affected joints whenever possible, but only within the limits of comfort. Range of motion should increase over time as you exercise regularly.

Walking is an excellent, low-impact, weight-bearing exercise that you can adjust to your individual physical abilities and limitations. Swimming is good for all-round full body movement; although it lacks the benefit of weight-bearing exercise.

One of the best activities you can do for arthritis is *rebound* exercise. Rebound exercise, or *rebounding* as it is often called, is simply jumping up and down on an *elastic surface*. Jumping on a trampoline is rebound exercise, as is jumping on a mini-tramp or *rebounder*. Skipping rope, however, is *not* rebound exercise because it is done on a hard surface, which puts a great deal of stress on the joints. For those with arthritis, I highly recommend using a small 36-inch (90 cm) diameter rebounder. They are convenient all-season exercise tools. They take up little space and they fit in any room so that you can exercise in a temperature controlled environment, regardless of the weather outside.

Unlike jogging or skipping rope, rebounding is very gentle on the joints. The springs of the rebounder absorb almost 90 percent of the impact as you land on the mat, so you don't experience the numbing jolt as your feet hit with each step. Rebounding is no more traumatic than walking. However, because of the up-and-down forces applied on the legs as you jump, it stimulates bone and tissue building to a far greater degree than walking. It gives the same strengthening benefits as jogging, without the trauma of hitting a hard surface. NASA scientists who have studied rebound exercise report that it is up to 68 percent more effective as a form of exercise than jogging. So not only is it gentler on the joints than jogging, it is more efficient too.

Rebounding provides all the benefits of weight bearing exercise without the trauma and danger of injury. One of the major benefits of weight bearing exercise is the effect it has on the bones. When the skeletal system is put under pressure, it responds like your muscles do by becoming stronger. Bone, like other living tissue, is constantly being broken down and rebuilt. Up to adulthood, bone building is more rapid than bone breakdown. At about the age of 30, bone breakdown outpaces the rebuilding, and the bones gradually become less dense. If bone breakdown proceeds too rapidly, we can develop osteoporosis. Weight bearing exercise can slow down and even reverse this process. Rebounding is an excellent exercise for building strong bones, even after the age of 30. "I had been losing bone before I began the rebounder," says Nina. "I got my bone density test results back the other day. In the last year I gained 4.8 percent density in my lower spine and 3 percent in my hips."

Another benefit of rebounding is that fluids in your joints are actively exchanged. Moving up and down on the rebounding mat causes the force of gravity to act on your body in such a way that your entire body is squeezed like a sponge with each bounce. You feel these forces when you are in an elevator. When you go up, you feel like a weight is pressing you down. When you go down in an elevator, it feels as if you are being pulled up. These same forces act on your joints while rebounding. Even though most of the work seems to be in your feet and legs, your entire body feels the force of gravity acting on it. As you bounce, the fluids in *all* of the joints of your body are squeezed and exercised. With every bounce, toxins are forced out of your joints and oxygenated, nutrition-rich fluids are pulled in, giving your joints a refreshing cleanse.

Rebounding is the only form of exercise that affects all of the joints in the body at the same time. With each bounce, *every* joint in your body—your finger joints, ankles, back, neck, shoulders—get exercised. You may accomplish about 100 bounces in a minute. If you rebound for just five minutes, you have worked each joint in your body a total of 500 times or repetitions. In 15 minutes you have done 1,500 reps! That's a lot of good movement and fluid exchange.

Rebounding is one exercise that virtually *anyone* can do no matter what their physical condition. Even those with severe physical limitations can rebound. The reason why is that each individual sets his or her own pace and level of intensity. If you are training for athletic competition you can intensify your workouts for maximum effect. If, on the other hand, you have a problem that limits what you can do, you can scale it back to your comfort level. Even if you are confined to a wheelchair you *can* rebound! In fact, many arthritis sufferers who have been confined to wheelchairs or walkers have used rebounding to regenerate their knees and ankles.

128

How can someone in a wheelchair jump on a mini-tramp, you might ask. There are several ways. If the person can stand, then she can stand on the mat. Stabilizing bars can be purchased that attach to the rebounder for the person to hold and maintain balance. You need not jump into the air, just bending the knees and flowing with the gentle swaying motion of the mat is enough to increase circulation into the knees and joints. In time, the joints will loosen and become stronger and more mobile. The height of the jumping can increase as the person feels able.

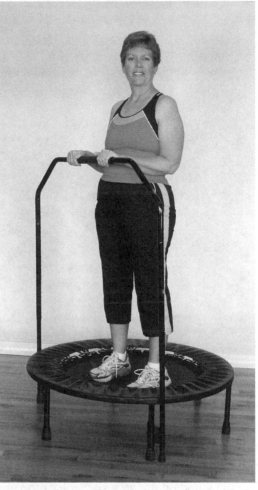

Rebounder with stabilizing bar to help maintain balance.

Another method is to simply sit down on the rebounder, with your rear end on the mat, knees over the edge, and feet on the floor. In this position, using your arms, you can gently bounce your torso and work your knees and ankles (see photo on next page).

One woman had rheumatoid arthritis so severe that she could not bend her stiffened knees more than a couple of inches, and was confined to a wheelchair. She was instructed to start rebounding daily. The way she did this was to wheel her chair up against the edge of

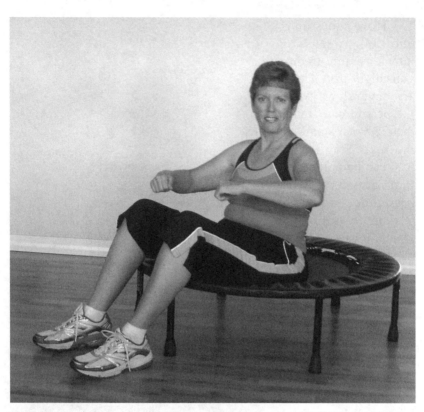

If arthritic knees prevent you from jumping on the rebounder, you can sit on the mat and bounce by moving your arms like a bird flapping its wings.

the rebounder, lift her feet, and rest them on top of the mat. Another person stood on the opposite side of the mat and gently bounced. The bounce was soft enough to cause her no discomfort. In time, as the circulation in her knees improved, the joints began to loosen up and the bouncing height was increased. As mobility in her knees improved, she was able to straighten out her legs and stand. She would come into the clinic on a walker, step up on the mat under her own power, and using a stabilizing bar, jump on her own. After several months, she progressed to the point that she was able to walk into the clinic without any assistance and get on the rebounder and jump. At one time she was destined to be confined to a wheelchair for the rest of her life, with no hope from conventional medicine for recovery. With rebound exercise she is now able to walk again and has regained her freedom.[6]

Thousands of people have discovered the healing benefits of rebound exercise simply by doing it. Dorothy had arthritis in her right knee and both ankles; bursitis in her right shoulder and both hips; suffered constant back aches; and was chronically fatigued. High blood pressure, frequent headaches, and poor balance plagued her as well. "All this had been going on for years on end," she says. "I was constantly under a doctor's care. He told me I was just getting old and had to expect this sort of thing."

One day Walt, Dorothy's husband, brought home a rebounder. "He was excited," she says, "but I was skeptical. For three days I watched him bounce for 30 seconds at a time. Each day he seemed brighter and had more energy. His disposition turned happy and sunny and he literally began to whistle while he worked, something I hadn't heard for a long time."

Encouraged by her husband's progress she decided to follow his example. "I tried to use the rebounder,' she said, "but couldn't keep my balance. Walt held my hands to steady me morning and evening for three days. Sure enough, I began to feel better too! In two weeks my blood pressure dropped 30 points! I had more stamina and I lost 8 pounds. I began to sing while I worked—literally sing! Life took on a whole new outlook. I had hurt and been tired for so long, I had actually forgotten how it felt to feel really good—no, really great! After just two and a half months, my back aches and headaches were gone. No more arthritis or bursitis pain. The leg and foot cramps that woke me up every night disappeared. I went from a size 24 to a size 18!"[7]

Rebounding is more than just a mode of exercise; it is a healing therapy that can affect the health of not only the joints, but the entire body.

The Best Time to Start is Now

Contrary to what some people seem to think, physical fitness is not a spectator sport! You need to get personally involved. Don't wait any longer. Start exercising now. If you don't have a rebounder, start walking, ride a bike, join a gym, become active.

If you are like most people, you don't exercise and probably aren't motivated to do it. Perhaps you've tried to establish an exercise program, but for one reason or another, you just couldn't stick to it. It is easy to be distracted or become discouraged and simply lose interest.

Most of us understand the need for exercise and want the benefits that come from it, but aren't motivated enough to stick with it or become discouraged easily. To make your exercise program successful, you need to make it a habit. Even if you have always avoided exercise, once you have made up your mind to do it and make it a habit, the psychological barriers will vanish and you will actually come to enjoy it. The following guidelines will help you set up and maintain a successful exercise program:

Make a Commitment

The first step is to make a commitment to yourself. Set a goal to exercise regularly. You should exercise a minimum of three times a week. Five to six days a week would be better.

Do Something You Can Enjoy

Select an activity you enjoy doing. The more you enjoy your workout, the more likely you are to make it a habit.

At Least 20 Minutes

Exercise at least 20 minutes at each session. Thirty minutes or more is even better. The more time you can spend, the more benefit you will receive.

Schedule Time to Exercise

You need to set a specific time to exercise and stick strictly to that schedule. This is very important! If you do not set aside a specific time for exercise, you will not keep it up. Other things always have a way of popping up, and before you know it, there is no time to exercise. Scheduling is a most important step in developing a successful exercise program. When you set a regular time to exercise, you adjust all other activities around your exercise schedule, so nothing else interferes. Having a set time will also psychologically prepare you for the workout. Before the habit is formed, you may argue with yourself after a hard day at work: "I'm too tired; I've got to make dinner; I've got to do this or do that." But if you have a schedule, it will encourage you to exercise regardless of the excuses.

Have a Place to Exercise

Choose a place to exercise and do it in the same place each time, a room in the house, the garage, a health club, or even outdoors. Your mind will associate this place with exercise, mentally you will feel more prepared, and your desire to exercise will increase. One reason some people prefer to exercise at health clubs is that the atmosphere helps get them into the mood.

Set Goals

Set goals for yourself and focus on accomplishing those goals. You should have at least two goals, one long-range and one short-range. The long-range goal would be to gain better joint and overall health. This is your primary purpose in initiating an exercise program. Short-range goals will be based on performance, such as time or distance. The short-range goals will make your workouts more enjoyable and give you feelings of accomplishment and progress. Make the goals realistic—not too easy, yet achievable in a matter of months. Once you have achieved one goal, set a new goal and go for it. Continue to set new goals as you accomplish old ones. Setting goals will give your workouts more purpose and will allow you to see the improvement you are making.

Become more physical in your everyday life. Don't limit your physical activity to just your regular exercise program. Take an opportunity to exercise whenever you can. Go bowling, take tennis lessons, go hiking, or get involved in other activities. Since exercise will make you more physically fit, take advantage of it. Instead of driving to a friend's house, walk or ride a bicycle. When you go to work, park your car at the far end of the lot and walk the rest of the way. Instead of taking the elevator, use the stairs. Take spontaneous walks outside. Go to the park and eat your lunch. Avoid sitting for extended periods. Get up and move about, move those joints and circulate that blood. When you rest, you rust. Motion is life.

133

Chapter 10

Lighten Your Load

Reduce the Stress on Your Joints

One of the things you can do right now to help ease the pain of arthritis is to lose some excess weight. Being overweight is a recognized risk factor for arthritis, especially osteoarthritis.[1]

The link between body weight and arthritis was first noticed in the 1960s. In a study conducted at Chicago's Cook County Hospital, doctors observed that obesity was common in osteoarthritis patients, and that a large percentage of them had gained weight just before the disease hit. Fifty percent of those with osteoarthritis had been overweight for only 3 to 10 years prior to the onset of the disease.[2]

Just 16 percent of normal weight adults report doctor diagnosed arthritis compared to 21.7 percent overweight and 30.6 percent obese adults. This is not surprising. Since excess body weight puts enormous strain on the joints, the pain and damage caused by osteoarthritis is intensified. Obesity can damage joints by forcing them to bear too much weight.

The knees and hips, which are the primary weight bearing joints of the body, handle loads from 2.5 to 10 times a person's body weight, depending on the joint. This means that if you weigh 200 pounds (90 kg), some of the joints may be handling as much as a ton (2,000 pounds/900 kg) of pressure as you walk, run, or otherwise use them. Every pound you carry puts an average of about five pounds (2.3 kg)

134

of added stress on your hips, knees, and ankles when you move. So, being just 10 pounds (4.5 kg) overweight is like having 50 extra pounds (23 kg) of pressure on your joints. Clearly, the load on your joints can become incredibly difficult to bear as your body weight increases.

Research shows that carrying even a little extra weight triples your chances of developing arthritis. Research also has shown, however, that for a woman of average height, losing as little as 11 pounds (5 kg) may cut the risk of osteoarthritis of the knee by up to 50 percent.

Even if you already have osteoarthritis, losing excess weight can help. When arthritis patients lose excess weight, arthritis symptoms can significantly improve.[3] In one study, researchers found that in patients with knee osteoarthritis, a weight reduction of 10 pounds improved function by 28 percent.[4] Every 10 pounds a person loses reduces the stress on the knees, hips, and ankles by 50 pounds. It is no wonder why weight loss improves joint health.

In addition to the excess strain placed on the joints, those who are overweight also tend to be less physically active. Thus their joints don't get needed movement to keep the joint tissue healthy. Less activity increases the risk of an infection taking up residence in joint tissue. Being overweight suggests poor eating habits. Foods that contribute most to weight gain (sugar and refined carbohydrates) are also those that encourage unfriendly bacteria growth in the mouth and digestive tract and depress the immune system. It is no wonder that overweight is a strong risk factor for arthritis.

Low-Fat Dieting Doesn't Work

Most overweight individuals don't like the excess weight and would prefer to be slimmer. Losing excess weight isn't always an easy matter. There is a big difference between wanting to lose weight and actually doing it.

Many people struggle endlessly to lose weight on low-fat, low-calorie diets of one sort or another. Unfortunately, most people fail. They may lose weight for a time, but as soon as they stop dieting the weight comes roaring back, often bringing along a few extra pounds for good measure. The dieter ultimately ends up weighing just as much or more then he or she did before going on the diet. A person may try again at a later date. At first she loses some weight but as soon as she stops dieting the cycle repeats itself. Over 90 percent of those people who go on weight loss diets ultimately regain all their lost weight.

These diets are failures. The reason they fail is that they are inherently designed to fail. Most weight loss diets are designed to restrict fat and calorie consumption. Fat is restricted because it contains twice as many calories per gram as protein or carbohydrate. The reasoning is that if you cut out fat, then you can eat twice as much of the other foods (protein or carbohydrate) for the same amount of calories. Therefore, it would be easier to reduce total calorie intake if you eliminate most of the fat.

In theory it sounds good, however, it doesn't work. There is one huge flaw in the low-fat concept of dieting. Fat has a remarkable ability to satisfy hunger. Fats slow down the digestive process, prompting the feeling of satisfaction sooner and maintaining it longer between meals. Carbohydrates (sugar, bread, grains, starchy foods), on the other hand, are digested very quickly so it takes more of them to feel full and hunger returns sooner after eating. Carbohydrate rich foods also affect blood sugar levels and stimulate hunger. What happens is that you end up eating many times more calories in carbohydrates as you would in fats, even though the fat, gram for gram, has more calories.

If, however, you restrict your carbohydrate consumption instead of the fat, you eat until you are satisfied and end up consuming fewer calories. A low-carb, moderate-fat diet is much more pleasant to handle and is vastly more filling on fewer calories. Weight loss is easier.

Coconut Oil for Weight Loss

The low-carb concept can be taken a step further if you use coconut oil as the primary source of fat in your diet. If you replace all other vegetable oils in the diet with coconut oil, your success at weight loss will be greatly enhanced. Coconut oil has special characteristics that support weight loss in a calorie restricted diet. One of the features that separates coconut oil from other fats and oils is that it is metabolized differently in the body than other fats. Unlike other fats, coconut oil is preferentially burned by the body to produce energy, rather than storing it as body fat. What this means is that when you eat coconut oil, little is stored as fat in the body; instead it is processed more like a carbohydrate and used to produce energy. Coconut oil is such an efficient source of energy that when the body burns it, it causes an immediate increase in metabolism. Your metabolism is actually kicked up a notch. Research has shown that after a single meal containing coconut oil, metabolism is elevated and is kept elevated for a full 24 hours! So for 24 hours, you have a higher level of energy and your body is burning calories at an accelerated rate. Therefore, more calories are burned off and fewer are left to be converted into body fat.

By utilizing the hunger satisfying and metabolism boosting effects of coconut oil, you can lose weight much more easily than you can on a low-fat diet. Researchers at McGill University in Canada have estimated that if you replace all the oils in your diet with a fat composed of medium-chain fatty acids, like coconut oil, you could lose up to 36 pounds (16 kg) a year![5] This is without dieting, without exercising, without changing the way you eat in any way, but by simply changing the type of oil you use.

Does this diet work? You bet it does! Rose Fenton says, "After taking a small amount of the virgin coconut oil every day for the last 3-4 months, I am now delighted to say that I have lost over 31 lbs in weight. I can hardly believe it, but I am now back to size 12 from being size 18 and feel so much better for it! Needless to say, I am absolutely hooked on the virgin coconut oil! I also have it with a jacket potato and a little sea-salt and it is absolutely delicious, and various other ways of including it in my diet."

Madeleine says, "I've been taking coconut oil now for two months. Why? Because I was desperate with my weight. I tried *everything!* All the fat burners that exist, name it and I tried it! With some of them the side effects were very strong. I also do exercise three times a week. Nothing was helping me. So I decided to meet a nutritionist and he made me take coconut oil. I take 5 teaspoons per day along with five little meals. I have to say that I am pretty impressed. I lost 15 pounds! Finally something that really works! I don't even want to think on how much money I spent on fat burners! I could have bought coconut oil for the rest of my life!"

"I didn't have many expectations when I started using coconut oil a year ago," says Sharon Maas. "I was overweight, and resigned to it; diets just didn't work with me." After learning about the benefits of coconut oil she replaced all the oils she had been using with coconut oil. The results were remarkable. "I lost 20 pounds in a matter of weeks, and what's more important, my weight has stayed at this level for the whole year. Even at times of more indulgence, such as holidays and Christmas. I did not gain. I take coconut oil with me wherever I go and can't live without my daily dose!"

Julie says, "I began taking 1 tablespoon of coconut oil before each meal on a 1,200 calorie diet. I have lost over 30 pounds over the past four months."

Suzzi says, "Currently I am taking a heaping tablespoon a day. I too have lost weight over the course of a year. I have lost 76 pounds and have been using the virgin coconut oil and eating mainly the Atkins diet with lots of veggies."

Danielle Johnson was on a waiting list for gastric bypass surgery when she learned about coconut oil. "I was a skeptic at first," she says, "but I opened up my mind to it because I'd tried so many other treatments for my obesity. I figured it was worth a shot…I've gone from tears and a life of despair over my weight, to a young, healthy vibrant 34-year-old. I feel as though I've captured my 20's once again. I have been using organic coconut oil for a week now and have lost 13 pounds! It's absolutely amazing. I weigh in at 360 pounds and was told by doctors that I would surely be at risk for heart disease and a host of other life threatening ailments due to my excess weight. I'd tried it all…Slim Fast, Nutrisystem, Weight Watchers, Atkins, South Beach, Relacore…you name it and I was out there buying it. I was just really desperate to find the answer to my life-long weight problem. I discovered through research and reading that the coconut cure along with spicy foods and organic foods, Yerba Mate Tea, and organic apple cider vinegar, would boost my metabolism through the roof and it *did!* It's only been a week and I'm running around here doing housework like a maniac and I can't sit still. My metabolism is so revved up and my cravings have totally vanished. I can't thank you enough for

138

renewing my faith in this wonderful thing we call life. I am shouting this information from the hilltops. The benefits are so tremendous that it's difficult not to broadcast it to all who will listen. I use the coconut oil as a moisturizer for my skin. I have no blemishes and my rosy cheeks have returned. I even buy the coconut powder and sprinkle it in my bath. It leaves my skin feeling soft and my psoriasis has literally disappeared. I no longer feel the aches and pains from fibromyalgia associated with my weight. I am a type II diabetic and my blood glucose levels have dropped significantly. I also noticed that the white powder on my feet that diabetics often get, has also disappeared. I can't say enough about this cure. It's not hocus pocus like some believe… I am quite certain that coconut oil will be in my life for always." What about the gastric bypass surgery she was waiting for? Danielle adds "I will no longer be needing it."

There is more to using coconut oil for weight loss than just adding the oil into the diet. Some people who already have a decent diet to begin with have reported that simply adding coconut oil to their meals stimulates weight loss. For the best results in losing excess weight, you should follow a low-carb regimen with coconut oil being the sole or primary fat in the diet. Eat 2 to 3 tablespoons of coconut oil daily, divided among each meal. Coconut oil helps to satisfy hunger so total calorie consumption should be monitored as well. Don't continue to eat the same size portions you have been in the habit of eating and then add the oil on top of that and expect to lose weight. Add the oil and reduce the total amount of other foods eaten. The oil will help curb your hunger so that you feel satisfied and don't get hungry between meals. "I have lost 55 pounds and still losing," says Zoe. "I'm never hungry and feel satisfied."

Another benefit of coconut oil is that it helps curb the cravings for sweets. Sugar is public enemy number one when it comes to weight loss (as well as tooth decay). Sugar is addictive much like a drug is. In fact, in animal studies where rats were given their choice between sugar and cocaine and had free access to each, guess what happened? The animals preferred the sugar over the cocaine.[6] This demonstrates the highly addictive nature and the enormous power of refined sugar. Another reason why most low-fat diets don't work is the fact that they allow too much sugar or sugar substitutes, which produce the same psychological reactions and dependence. It doesn't matter that these artificial sweeteners don't have many calories, the foods they are usually consumed with often do. Artificial sweeteners keep the fire of sugar cravings alive and active. A person cannot take control of her eating habits if she is controlled by cravings.

Adopting a whole foods diet is good for your health and helps you slim down. The low-carb whole foods diet described in Chapter 7 is the quickest and easiest way to lose excess weight. When combined with coconut oil, the weight loss is enhanced.

Most people who don't have the best diets to begin with may need a little more guidance. For these people I recommend my book *Eat Fat, Look Thin*. This book explains exactly how to use coconut oil to boost energy, stimulate metabolism, stop food cravings, and lose excess weight. It also describes the foods that are the biggest troublemakers and the foods that help you lose weight.

How to Use Coconut Oil

For weight loss, I recommend consuming 2 to 3 tablespoons of coconut oil daily. Ideally, the oil should be consumed with meals, a little at each meal to help satisfy hunger and prevent overeating. The simplest way to do this is to prepare your foods using the oil.

Coconut oil is very heat stable, so it is excellent for use in the kitchen. Use it for any baking or frying purpose. In recipes that call for margarine, butter, shortening, or vegetable oil, use coconut oil instead. Use the same amount or more to make sure you get the recommended amount in your diet.

Not all foods are prepared using oil, but you can still incorporate the oil into the diet. You can add coconut oil to foods that aren't normally prepared with oil. For example, add a spoonful of coconut oil to hot beverages (tea, coffee, milk), hot cereals, soups, sauces, casseroles, or use as a topping over cooked vegetables. A wonderful resource of recipes and cooking ideas is the book the *Coconut Lover's Cookbook*. It was written specifically to show how to incorporate coconut oil into the diet. It contains nearly 450 recipes ranging from salad dressings to beverages, soups, chowders, sauces, and main dishes.

Although I recommend that you consume the coconut oil with foods, you don't have to prepare your food with it or add it to the food. You can take it by the spoonful like a dietary supplement. Many people prefer to get their daily dose of coconut oil this way. If you use a good quality coconut oil, it tastes good. Many people don't like the thought of putting a spoonful of oil, any oil, into their mouths. It may take some people a little time to get used to it.

There are two primary types of coconut oil you will find sold in stores. One is called *virgin* coconut oil, the other is refined, bleached, and deodorized (RBD) coconut oil. Virgin coconut oil is made from fresh coconuts with very minimal processing. The oil basically comes straight from the coconut. Since it has gone through little processing, it retains a delicate coconut taste and aroma. It is delicious.

RBD coconut oil is made from copra or dried coconut and has gone through more extensive processing. During the processing all the flavor and aroma have been removed. For people who don't like the taste of coconut in their foods, this is a good option. RBD oil is processed using mechanical means and high temperatures. Chemicals are not generally used. When you go to the store, you can tell the difference between virgin and RBD coconut oils by the label. All virgin coconut oils will state that they are "virgin." RBD oils will not have this statement. They also do not say "RBD." Sometimes they will be advertised as "Expeller Pressed," which means that the initial pressing of the oil from the coconut meat was done mechanically, without the use of heat. However, heat is usually used at some later stage of the refining process.

Many people prefer the virgin coconut oil because it has undergone less processing and retains more of the nutrients and the flavor that nature put into it. This is why it maintains its coconut flavor. Because more care is taken to produce virgin coconut oil, it is more expensive than RBD oil.

Most brands of RBD oil are generally tasteless and odorless and differ little from each other. The quality of the different brands of virgin coconut oil, however, can vary greatly. There are many different processing methods used to produce virgin coconut oil. Some are better than others. Plus, the care taken also affects the quality. Some companies produce excellent quality coconut oil that tastes so good,

141

you can easily eat it off the spoon. Other brands are strongly flavored and unpalatable. You cannot tell the difference just by looking at the jar. You have to taste it. If the oil has a mild coconut flavor with a mild coconut smell and tastes good to you, then that is a brand you should use. If the flavor is overpowering or smells smoky, you might want to try another brand.

Coconut oil is available at all health food stores and many grocery stores, as well as on the Internet. There are many different brands to choose from. Generally the more expensive brands are the best quality, but not always. The cheaper brands of virgin coconut oil are almost always of inferior quality. All brands, however, have basically the same culinary and therapeutic effects and are useful.

If you purchase coconut oil from the store, it may have the appearance of shortening, being firm and snow white in color. When you take it home and put it on your kitchen shelf, after a few days it may transform into a colorless liquid. Don't be alarmed. This is natural. One of the distinctive characteristics of coconut oil is its high melting point. At temperatures of 76 degrees F (24 C) and above, the oil is liquid like any other vegetable oil. At temperatures below this level, it solidifies. It is much like butter. If stored in the refrigerator, a stick of butter is solid, but let it sit on the countertop on a hot day and it melts into a puddle. A jar of coconut oil may be liquid or solid depending on the temperature where it is stored. You can use it whether it is solid or liquid.

Coconut oil is very stable so it does not need to be refrigerated. You can store it on a cupboard shelf. Shelf life for a good quality coconut oil is 1 to 3 years. Hopefully, you would use it long before then.

Chapter 11

Inflammation Busters

More than 200 drugs, including NSAIDs, corticosteroids, gold salts, and anti-rheumatic drugs, are used in the treatment of arthritis. None of these drugs has been found safe; all are known to produce mild to serious side effects.[1] Long term use increases the risk. NSAIDs alone kill some 30,000 people every year. They are also linked to circulation problems and heart failure; Vioxx and Celebrex are prime examples of the very real dangers of drug use. These two NSAIDs, used to treat arthritis, have caused numerous deaths from heart attacks and strokes.

There are, however, natural substances that can reduce inflammation, swelling, and pain without adverse side effects. These substances are foods or food components that have been used safely for thousands of years. While these foods will not cure arthritis (but neither can the drugs), they can help to temporarily ease the pain without causing further harm.

Omega-3 Essential Fatty Acids

There are two classes of essential fatty acids: omega-3s and omega-6s. The best known omega-3 oils are flaxseed and fish oils. The omega-6 oils include most of the vegetables oils we see in the grocery store—corn, soybean, safflower, etc.

Omega-3s and omega-6 oils produce hormone-like chemicals called prostaglandins. The prostaglandins produced by omega-3 oils have an opposite effect to those produced by omega-6 oils. For instance, prostaglandins from omega-3 oils have an anti-inflammatory effect, while those from omega-6 oils have pro-inflammatory effects. If you have arthritis, getting an adequate amount of omega-3s in your diet can help calm inflammation and ease pain. On the other hand, consuming omega-6 oils will intensify the inflammation and pain. This is one of the reasons why I don't recommend eating processed vegetable oils.

Omega-3 and omega-6 oils are considered *essential* because our bodies can't make them from other nutrients. So we must get them from our diets. Our need for both oils is rather small, only a few grams a day. We need both in our diet, which is why they are called essential fatty acids. Since these oils have competing and opposing actions, they need to be consumed in balance. In the process of making prostaglandins, both essential fatty acids compete with one another for the body's enzyme reserves. Too much of one will prevent the synthesis of the other. So, excessively high intakes of one will create a deficiency of the other.

We hear a lot about not getting adequate amounts of omega-3 oils; that is because there are far fewer sources of this fat than there are for omega-6. Omega-6 fatty acids are found everywhere. Almost all foods contain omega-6 fatty acids—vegetables, grains, meats, fish, eggs, milk, nuts, seeds—in fact, it is hard to find foods that do not contain omega-6 fatty acids. The richest source of omega-6 fatty acids are processed vegetable oils. They can contain as much as 80 percent omega-6. When you look at how much vegetable oils are used in food processing these days, you will understand why we consume between 10 and 20 times as much omega-6 as we do omega-3. This has caused a general omega-3 deficiency in our society.

To correct the problem, we don't necessarily need to add a bunch of omega-3 fatty acids supplements into our diet, but we can accomplish the same goal simply by cutting out processed vegetable oils. This would do a tremendous amount of good in balancing our total essential fatty acid intake.

A problem we have with omega-3 oils is that they are very delicate and oxidize (go rancid) easily. Once extracted from their source, oxidation begins. Oxidation causes the formation of harmful free radicals. Therefore, omega-3 oils must be consumed as fresh as possible. Many omega-3 oils in dietary supplements are already going rancid before they even leave the store, especially if they were not refrigerated. All omega-3 dietary supplements should be refrigerated to retard oxidation.

The best way to get your omega-3s is not from dietary supplements but directly from food, just as our ancestors did. Eating omega-3 rich foods insures that the oil is fresh and not rancid. The best food sources are fish and eggs laid by free-range chickens (chickens that are able to roam around and eat freely). The fat in grass-fed beef also supplies omega-3s. Grass is a rich source of omega-3s, and when cattle eat the grass their own tissues are enriched with this oil. Plant sources of omega-3 include seaweed, green leafy vegetables (beet greens, chard, spinach, bok choy, etc.), and flaxseed.

Gram for gram, animal sources are almost 10 times more potent or effective as the plant sources. The reason for this is that the omega-3s in animal sources are easily utilized by our bodies to make prostaglandins, which is their primary biological function. The omega-3s in plant sources need to be synthesized into a form that matches the type found in animals. This process takes many steps and only about 10 percent of the original plant derived omega-3 is completely converted in the usable animal form.

Turmeric: A Taste of India

Have you eaten a good curry lately? If so, you've upped your protection against arthritis as well as indigestion, free-radical damage, heart disease, and cancer. The secret is turmeric—the spice that gives curry its bright, gold-yellow color.

Turmeric is made from the underground stalk of the *Curcuma longa* plant. In India it is used not only as a flavoring, but for the preservation of food and as a yellow dye for textiles. It is an important element of Ayurvedic medicine, where it is used to treat a variety of health problems including arthritis, wounds, skin problems, ulcers, colitis, and other inflammatory diseases. The success of this spice in traditional medicine has encouraged researchers to investigate its therapeutic potential.

145

Much of turmeric's medicinal properties come from curcumin, the yellow pigment that gives the spice its distinctive color. Extensive research over the past two decades has shown that curcumin exerts potent anti-inflammatory action.[2] In addition, curcumin also exhibits antioxidant, antiviral, antibacterial, antifungal, and anticancer activities and thus has potential against various malignant diseases.[3]

Because of its potent anti-inflammatory effects, researchers are recommending it as a natural and harmless treatment for arthritis and other inflammatory diseases. In addition to calming inflammation, turmeric also spices up your immune system and increases your ability to fight off infection. Curcumin has been shown to activate the white blood cells that protect us against microscopic invaders and to enhance antibody response. This combined with the antimicrobial effects gives our immune system a defensive boost to fight off chronic infection. So turmeric provides a double benefit for arthritis sufferers.

Recent research has discovered another compound in turmeric that may have a greater anti-inflammatory effect than curcumin. It is referred to as turmeric oil. Eating turmeric provides both curcumin and turmeric oil.

The best way to get the benefits of curcumin and turmeric oil is by using turmeric in your cooking. Add it to soups, sauces, steamed vegetables, casseroles, and even sprinkle it on meats, fish, and chicken. If you don't like using this spice in every meal, you can also purchase turmeric dietary supplements. These supplements have proven to "profoundly inhibit joint inflammation and periarticular joint destruction" in arthritic joints.[4] Dietary supplements of turmeric are available in tablets and capsules. For arthritis, Dr. Andrew Weil, MD recommends 400 to 600 mg of turmeric extract, taken three times a day with foods.

Because of turmeric's anti-inflammatory, antimicrobial, and immune boosting properties, it can be a valuable aid in overcoming arthritis. In amounts typically used for culinary purposes it is believed to provide beneficial effects in treating other health problems as well including allergies, asthma, heart disease, Alzheimer's disease, diabetes, and cancer.[5] Because of its venerable value in Ayurvedic medicine, as well as its many newly discovered therapeutic uses, turmeric is fittingly referred to as the "Spice for Life."

Ginger: Another Gift from India

Ginger is another popular spice in Indian cookery. When you smell the fragrance of Indian cooking you can't help but savor the aroma of ginger. Ginger comes from the underground stem or rhizome of the plant *Zingiber officinale*. Because of its appearance it is called the "horn root" in Indian Sanskrit. It has been used in medicine in Asian, Indian, and Arabic herbal traditions since ancient times. In Asia, ginger has been used for more than 2,000 years to treat stomach upset, nausea, colic, diarrhea, and as an aid to digestion. Most of the research to date has focused on its ability to ease nausea and vomiting caused by motion sickness, morning sickness during pregnancy, and other conditions.

In addition to settling the stomach and improving digestive function, ginger also exhibits anti-inflammatory action and is being used to treat arthritis, ulcerative colitis, and other inflammatory conditions. Studies validate the use of ginger as an aid for those with arthritis. In a study of 261 people with osteoarthritis of the knee, those who received a ginger extract twice daily experienced less pain and required fewer painkilling medications compared to those who received a placebo.[6]

In another study, 56 patients (28 with rheumatoid arthritis, 18 with osteoarthritis, and 10 with muscular discomfort) used powdered ginger in their foods. Among the arthritis patients, more than three-quarters experienced, to varying degrees, relief in pain and swelling. All the patients with muscular discomfort experienced relief in pain. None of the participants reported any adverse effects during the period of ginger consumption, which ranged from 3 months to 2½ years.[7]

The active ingredient in ginger that imparts its distinctive flavor and its medicinal value is a volatile oil known as *gingerol*. Chemically, gingerol is very similar to capsaicin, the compound that gives chili peppers their bite. Fresh ginger, like chili pepper, adds a spicy "heat" to foods. Gingerol works its magic on arthritis by inhibiting the formation of chemicals that trigger inflammation.

Ginger is available as a powdered spice, liquid extract, or fresh root. The powdered form is convenient to use in cooking, but the fresh root has a pleasant lemony flavor that can't be matched by the powdered form. Ginger tea is simple to make. Put a few thinly sliced pieces of fresh ginger into 8 ounces of boiling water. Let it simmer for a few minutes, remove from heat, let it cool, remove the ginger, add a touch of honey, and enjoy.

A few drops of ginger oil mixed with a little coconut oil can be rubbed into arthritic joints to help ease pain. You could also make a poultice or compress with fresh or powdered ginger and place it over the affected joint.

For those who just don't like the taste of ginger or don't want it in their foods, you could also use ginger capsules. Follow the recommendations on the label.

Cherries for Gout

Have joint pain? Eat a bowl of cherries. Believe it or not, cherries can help relieve the pain of gout and other forms of arthritis. Fighting the effects of arthritis may never have tasted so good.

Back in the 1940s Dr. Ludwig W. Blau accidentally discovered that cherries can relieve the pain associated with gout. Dr. Blau suffered with gout himself. His condition was so severe that he was confined to a wheelchair. Since cherry season is short, he took advantage of the opportunity one day by feasting on a large bowl of the fresh fruit. The following day, to his surprise, the pain in his feet was gone. Since he hadn't done anything different than usual, except eating the cherries, he suspected that they were the cause of his good fortune. He continued eating a minimum of six cherries (fresh, dried, or frozen) every day and remained pain free and was able to leave his wheelchair for good and lead a normal life. Dr. Blau began recommending cherries to other gout patients who also experienced similar results.

The first study to test Dr. Blau's ideas was performed in the 1950s and involved 12 individuals with gout. The study confirmed that eating a half-pound of cherries or the equivalent amount of cherry juice prevented gout attacks. Black, sweet yellow, and red sour cherries were all effective. Since that time, several other studies have confirmed these results. These studies show that cherry consumption lowers blood levels of urate, the primary building block of sodium urate crystals that collect in gout-affected joints.[8]

148

Cherries are not only beneficial for relieving the symptoms associated with gout, but can be of benefit for all arthritis sufferers. Cherries are a rich source of antioxidant nutrients such as vitamin C. They also contain a group of potent antioxidants called *anthocyanins*. These antioxidants not only block the progression of free radicals, but also extinguish the fire of inflammation. Studies show that anthocyanins effectively lower arthritic inflammation and swelling.[9-10]

Virtually all types of cherries are effective, both sweet and sour. Strawberries, blueberries, and other berries may also be beneficial because they too are rich sources of antioxidants and appear to also have anti-inflammation action.[11]

Tropical Fruits

Eating a bowl of fresh, juicy tropical fruit not only tastes delicious but may also help calm the inflammation in your joints. Several tropical fruits, namely pineapple, papaya, kiwi, mango, figs, and guava contain special protein-digesting enzymes that apparently can also help ease inflammation.[12-14]

Among these, pineapple has received the greatest attention and study. Back in 1956 a Philadelphia dentist reported that bromelain, the protein digesting enzyme in pineapple, diminished pain and swelling in his patients suffering from multiple dental impactions.[15]

The protein digestive enzymes in pineapple and other tropical fruits have become popular as commercial meat tenderizers and as digestive aids. Approximately 90 percent of the meat tenderizers used in consumer households contain bromelain. It is sold as a powder or combined with marinade to be used on uncooked meat. The enzyme penetrates the meat, breaking down the protein, making it tender when cooked. Bromelain is deactivated when heated, so the tenderizing occurs before the meat is cooked.

Because it breaks down protein, bromelain is commonly used as a digestive aid to help the stomach digest the protein in foods. A slice of fresh pineapple makes an excellent digestive aid to accompany high protein meals. Cooked or canned pineapple, however, has no digestive benefit.

149

Bromelain was first reported to be of value for relieving pain and reducing inflammation for use in both rheumatoid arthritis and osteoarthritic patients in 1964.[16] Studies since that time have confirmed bromelain's anti-inflammatory action.[17]

Bromelain has become very popular as an effective alternative to NSAIDs. In Germany it is approved by the Commission E for the treatment of inflammation and swelling and is one of the most widely used herbal medicines in that country.

When used as a digestive aid, bromelain is usually taken with meals. When used for inflammatory conditions, it is taken on an empty stomach to maximize absorption into the bloodstream.

Bromelain has been used in daily dosages ranging from 200 to 2000 mg, with therapeutic action shown at only 160 mg/day. Doses between 200 and 400 mg a day over a period of one month have shown to be beneficial for treating arthritis.

Fruits and Vegetables

A variety of vitamins, minerals, antioxidants and other phytonutrients are found in virtually all fresh fruits and vegetables, herbs, and spices; many of which help to ease inflammation, fight against destructive free radicals, boost the immune system, and aid in strengthening and building strong bones and joint tissues. Researchers have yet to identify all the potential anti-inflammatory substances in fresh foods. Some of the more thoroughly researched include reservatrol (red grapes, cranberries, tomatoes, and peanuts), quercetin (onions and apples), silymarin (artichokes), cyanidin 3-glucoside (mulberries), and luteolin (celery and green peppers).[18-20] Several preclinical and clinical studies suggest that these agents have potential for arthritis treatment.

Simply incorporating an ample variety of fresh fruits and vegetables into your daily diet can help deliver many health-building, arthritis-fighting nutrients. Studies have repeatedly shown the benefits of fruit and vegetable consumption. We should follow the advice from the U.S. Department of Health and Human Resources, and consume five or more servings of fruits and vegetables daily. This is a minimum. We should actually consume more and push out other, less healthy foods from our diet.

Chapter 12

The Arthritis Battle Plan

Seven Steps to Beating Arthritis and Fibromyalgia

You can win the war against arthritis and fibromyalgia. In this chapter, each step in the battle plan is laid out. The following briefly summarizes the steps you need to take. Details of each step are covered in previous chapters.

Step 1: Oral Health

In addition to your normal, daily dental hygiene routine, you should add oil pulling. Every morning, before breakfast and before brushing your teeth, swish about 2 teaspoons of coconut oil in your mouth. Work the oil around your teeth and gums vigorously. Do this for 15 to 20 minutes. You can read, use the computer, prepare for the day, or do most any other task while oil pulling to keep from getting bored and to make good use of your time.

If you have active tooth decay or gum disease or if your arthritis is causing a lot of trouble, you may want to increase the number of times you oil pull to 2 or 3 times a day. Pull on an empty stomach, just before meals is a good time. As you feel better, you can reduce the number of times you pull to once daily.

If you have serious dental issues, you need to visit your dentist and get them taken care of. Think carefully before having any root canal procedure performed.

Step 2: Fight Systemic Infection

To help fight an active infection in your body, consume 3 to 4 tablespoons of coconut oil daily. Once the infection is under control, you can reduce this to 1 to 3 tablespoons daily as a maintenance dose. You can eat the oil anytime, but it is preferable with foods at mealtime. You can use the oil in food preparation or can take it by the spoonful.

There are no harmful side effects to eating coconut oil, however, if you are not accustomed to eating much oil in your diet, suddenly adding the oil may loosen your bowels somewhat. So, you may want to start off taking only 1 tablespoon daily for the first week or two and gradually build up to more.

Step 3: Anti-Arthritis Diet

This is the most important step you can take in overcoming arthritis. The more diligent you are in following this diet, the better your chances are for success.

Focus on eating a healthy diet composed of *fresh* fruits, vegetables, whole grains, nuts, seeds, meats, eggs, and dairy, preferably organically grown or raised. Avoid sugar, sweets, refined grain products, and processed vegetable oils as much as possible. Reduce or eliminate processed, packaged foods. If the food has been cooked and is sold in a can, box, plastic, or other container, it is best to leave it alone. Any commercially prepared food that lists several items on the ingredient label and includes multisyllabic words you find difficult to pronounce, is best not eaten.

Work toward a goal of preparing your meals using at least 90 percent fresh ingredients. The remaining portion can come from commercially prepared foods, most of which would be condiments and incidental food items and contain no harmful chemical additives.

Sugar and sugar-sweetened foods are your biggest enemies. They feed disease-causing microbes in your mouth, depress your immune system, provide little nutrition, and promote weight gain. The most important thing you can do to fight off arthritis is to eliminate sweets and highly refined grains, which are nearly as bad as sugar.

For help in adjusting your diet and learning how to eat naturally, follow the Seven-Day Whole Foods Challenge in the Appendix. Also, visit the websites of the Weston A. Price Foundation at www.westonaprice.org and the Price-Pottenger Nutrition Foundation at www.ppnf.org for information and resources.

Step 4: Joint Rejuvenation

To aid in joint rejuvenation and healing, you can take a dietary supplement containing the combination of glucosamine sulfate and chondroitin sulfate. The supplement should contain 1,500 mg of glucosamine sulfate and 1,200 mg of chondroitin sulfate per serving. Take one serving daily. A serving may consist of two or three capsules. Glucosamine/chondroitin is sold in health food stores and pharmacies.

Step 5: Exercise

Start an exercise program and stick to it. It need not be strenuous or expensive. Walking and swimming are good. Rebound exercise is ideal. Exercise at least three days a week for a minimum of 20 minutes a day, to start. Increase your time and days as you get stronger. One hour daily, five to six days a week is a good goal to shoot for.

Step 6: Weight Management

If you are overweight, losing a few extra pounds can make a significant difference in the way you feel. Utilize the metabolic boosting and hunger satisfying effects of coconut oil to help you lose excess weight. For best results with weight loss, follow a low-carb whole foods diet with coconut oil being your primary source of fat.

Step 7: Calm Inflammation

Incorporate into your diet foods and dietary supplements that help soothe the inflammation. This includes turmeric, ginger, cherries, and omega-3 fatty acids. Fish, seaweed, eggs, and leafy green vegetables provide a natural source of omega-3 fatty acids. A dietary supplement consisting of 200 to 400mg of bromelain taken on an empty stomach may also help. And finally, eat plenty of fresh fruits and vegetables to get a rich source of antioxidant nutrients. This step alone does not cure inflammation, but it can help. For permanent relief you need to focus on all the previous steps.

By following the Arthritis Battle Plan you can eliminate or significantly reduce the pain of arthritis and fibromyalgia. Does this program work? Just ask Barbara Moody. She had been active all her life. She jogged regularly and was an avid rock climber. Ten years ago she began to experience chronic pain that eventually affected her feet, knees, and back. The pain became so intense that it ended her active lifestyle and caused her to give up her career as a firefighter. Severe osteoarthritis in her vertebrae led to four back surgeries, one of which involved the fusion of two of her vertebrae. She tried to exercise regularly and participated in low-impact aerobics, but afterward she would often limp home in pain. The drugs her doctor prescribed were of little help, and her condition continued to deteriorate. Her doctors recommended that she have a fifth spine surgery and second fusion.

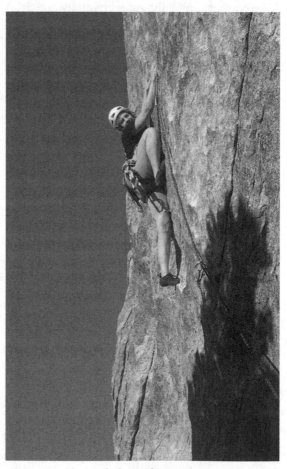

She learned about oil pulling and the benefits of coconut oil and began pulling faithfully every day and added the oil into her diet. Within a short time she began to notice some remark-

At age 60 and free from arthritis pain, Barbara is back scaling mountains again.

154

able changes taking place. Her teeth became noticeably whiter. The coating on her tongue was eliminated. Her loose gums tightened up around her teeth. Severe gingivitis, which had formed around the titanium post of a dental implant, healed up and about a quarter of an inch of her loosened gum was restored tightly around that molar.

In addition to her improved dental health, her physical health took a dramatic turn for the better. Within weeks the pain from osteoarthritis in her knees subsided. She was able to walk several miles without knee pain and to go up and down stairs without problem. She began rock climbing again.

Her recovery was documented thoroughly by her doctors, who were amazed at her sudden improvement after 10 years of chronic pain and disability. They told her she no longer needed back surgery. Impressed with her remarkable progress, three of her doctors are now oil pulling themselves, just to improve their general health.

Barb says this program "has truly changed my health and changed my life...I feel better than I have in years. I am 60 years old and have the energy I had when I was in my 30's."

Cleansing Reactions

One of the things you may experience as you begin this program is some heavy cleansing. Oil pulling and consuming coconut oil can each create a very dramatic cleansing or detoxifying reaction in some people.

One of the most common reactions with oil pulling is a heavy discharge of mucus. Oil pulling stimulates cleansing in the throat and sinuses. Consequently, mucus flow may increase. Some people experience this the first time they try oil pulling. Don't worry, this is a normal reaction. The body is expelling the mucus to purge toxins. You want these poisons out of your body. Over time, as toxins are cleansed from your system, mucus flow decreases.

Consuming coconut oil regularly can also bring on cleansing symptoms. Since the medium-chain fatty acids in the oil kill microbes, it can cause what doctor's refer to as a Herxheimer or "die off" reaction. The Herxheimer reaction may involve a variety of symptoms that are often mistaken for the flu, such as chills, fever, body aches,

155

headaches, rashes, nausea, vomiting, diarrhea, fatigue, etc. These symptoms aren't caused by an infection or disease, but occur as a result of therapies that kill infectious organisms in the body. They are not side effects of the therapy, but are evidence of the effectiveness of the therapy and the existence of an infection. The symptoms are caused by the release of toxins from dying organisms and the accumulation of dead bacteria. In response to this accumulation of garbage, the body shifts into a heightened stage of internal cleansing and detoxification to purge these poisons. Consequently, the reactions can be pronounced and mimic an illness. Taking antibiotics or drugs will be of no benefit and are discouraged as they may actually interfere with the cleansing process.

The cleansing reaction normally only lasts a few days, but may continue for as long as three weeks or more. The reaction may occur at any time you begin the program. It can happen almost immediately or weeks later. The types of symptoms you may encounter and their intensity varies from person to person. So you cannot compare your reaction with that of another person's. In some people, symptoms may be severe, while for others they may be so mild that the effects go entirely unnoticed. *Arthritis symptoms may intensify for a period of time* as toxins are released into the blood from the dying bacteria. Don't be surprised that your symptoms may get worse for a time before they get better.

This period of cleansing is also referred to as a *healing crisis*. During a healing crisis, refrain from taking any medications, unless they are required by your doctor. Drink plenty of water to assist the body in flushing the toxins from the body. If you don't feel like eating, don't, but you should get plenty of fluids. Cut back on heavy physical activity and get ample rest. Stay home from work if you need to. Continue oil pulling and eating the coconut oil.

Cleansing is an ongoing process so you may experience more than one healing crisis. Barbara, whose story was told above, describes her experience with cleansing, "About three days into oil pulling I experienced a mild sore throat that lasted only a day. Beginning at about 14 days into the process and over about a ten day period I coughed up close to 2 tablespoons daily full of thick sticky yellow mucus that became increasingly lighter and less viscous until it was just white. At about 10 weeks I had the 'mother of all healing crises' with 55 hours of fever that must have been hovering around 105 degrees at its highest. I knew that it was a healing crisis and that it would pass. I remember times of just sobbing I hurt so much. But at the same time I kept thinking that I must be burning out some pretty nasty stuff." Not everyone goes through as severe a crisis as Barbara did, but you should be aware that it can happen.

You don't need to be afraid of a healing crisis. It is a good thing and signals a period of cleansing and healing. After the cleanse is over, you will feel better than you have for a long time and have a heightened sense of well-being.

I Still Have Pain. What Do I Do?

What happens if, after following the Arthritis Battle Plan, you still experience joint pain? The problem may be that you have not given the program enough time to work. Many of us are too impatient; we plant a tomato seed in the morning and expect to pick ripened tomatoes in the afternoon. You need to give the seed time to grow. After planting, it may take a couple of weeks before you see anything at all happen. Then finally you will notice a small tender sprout gently poking its head up out of the soil. In time it grows bigger and more noticeable and finally it produces fruit. Your progress on this program is like the tomato seed. At first you may not notice much, but give it time. As the body repairs and heals itself, you will gradually notice changes. Just like you can't see a tomato plant grow inch by inch, you won't notice the gradual changes being made in your body either. But one day you will notice that you are doing things you hadn't been able to do for years, such as opening a tight jar lid or walking up the stairs without pain.

You may have had arthritis or fibromyalgia for years. The process that led up to your current condition may have taken 10 or 20 or more years to develop. So you can't expect to reverse all those years of degeneration in just a few short days or weeks. You need to allow time for your body to heal itself.

Every person's response will be different. You may experience noticeable improvement within a matter of days or weeks and continue to improve for some time. For others the process may take many months. This is a gradual process. So don't expect miracles to happen overnight. Some damage may be irreversible. If your joints are severely damaged (as shown on page 49), you can only expect a partial improvement, but even then, a partial improvement is better than none at all.

Not all joint pain is caused by arthritis. Another reason why you may not experience the results you desire might be because you do not have arthritis. Have you been diagnosed by a physician as having one of the various forms of arthritis? I am not talking about an off-hand comment from the doctor that you have "arthritis" but an official diagnosis such as rheumatoid arthritis, osteoarthritis, or ankylosing spondylitis? Or are you self-diagnosing based simply on the presence of pain? Just because you have pain in or near a joint doesn't mean you have arthritis. There are many conditions that can cause pain that aren't technically arthritis. Joint injuries are often mistaken as arthritis. Bursitis, tendonitis, and osteoporosis are common examples. This is why an exact diagnosis from a physician is useful.

The primary reason why people don't get the results they want is that they don't follow the program. Are you eating a whole foods diet? This is perhaps the biggest stumbling block to success with this plan. People often rationalize to themselves that a complete whole foods diet is unnecessary, that simply adding a few fresh fruits into the diet is good enough—it isn't. If you eat sweets and refined grains and add an apple and banana to your diet, you won't see any improvement. You need to eliminate or at least severely limit devitalized foods and replace them with nutritious whole foods. Eating a poor diet is the reason people develop arthritis in the first place. Refined carbohydrates especially feed the bacteria in our mouths that lead to oral infections, which in turn cause joint infections. In addition, poor nutrition lowers your body's ability to fight off infection. In order to reverse arthritis, you need to correct your diet. If you are still experiencing joint pain, the most likely reason is because of your diet. Go to the Appendix and take the Seven-Day Whole Foods Challenge to help you learn more about whole foods.

Are you oil pulling daily as directed? Do you have any dental issues that have not been resolved? Do you have root canals or crowns? These can be harboring infection. Even in the absence of any pain or noticeable symptoms, you could have a low-grade infection. The absence of pain is not necessarily an indication that there is no infection present. Go to the dentist for a check-up and have X-rays taken. If you need dental work, get it done. Sometimes people with serious dental problems hesitate to get the dental care they need, and as long as they don't experience pain, they put off getting treatment. This is a big mistake. Dental infections don't usually heal up by themselves. You must make an effort to correct the problem, either through dietary changes, oil pulling, better dental hygiene, or getting dental treatment, and usually all of the above.

Finally, not all cases of arthritis result from dental infections. Other tissues in the body could be acting as a focus of infection, spewing out bacteria and toxins that continually aggravate your joints. You need to locate these areas. Where might they be? The lungs, sex organs, urinary tract, and digestive tract are other sites of infection. Have you had problems in the past in any of these areas? Have you had asthma or bronchitis? Venereal disease? Frequent urinary tract infections or kidney stones? Digestive troubles, colitis, diverticulitis, candidiasis, or parasites?

The gastrointestinal tract is a potential source of infection. Like the mouth, our intestines are the home to many microorganisms, some of which can cause a great deal of trouble if they get into the bloodstream. Ulcers, diverticuli, permeable gut (leaky gut syndrome), parasites, and other conditions can be spreading infection into the bloodstream. In this case, you need to work on improving the health of your digestive system and the microbial environment within it. Food allergies could also be contributing to the problem.

For better digestive health follow the diet described in this book, identify and eliminate all foods that cause allergies or sensitivities, and use coconut oil regularly. Dietary measures usually take time. So give your body the time it needs to heal. A resource that may help you achieve this goal is *The Body Ecology Diet* by Donna Gates. This book describes how to establish and nourish the growth of beneficial microorganisms in the digestive tract and suppress the growth of harmful ones.

You Can Achieve Success

Following the Seven Steps to Beating Arthritis and Fibromyalgia can have a dramatic impact on your life. I receive letters and emails from readers all over the world who share their experiences. I would like to share one from a woman who was diagnosed with chronic fatigue syndrome and fibromyalgia. I'll let her tell her own story.

My name is Jo Wilkinson, I'm 39 and live in the UK. In 1987 I was diagnosed with what was then called Post Viral Syndrome, now ME/CFS/CFIDS [chronic fatigue syndrome and fibromyalgia]. I'd had a serious bout of flu in 1986 from which I did not recover properly, although my health had been slowly deteriorating since mid 1985. I had a severe relapse in 1993 following a flu vaccination. From this point I was often house and/or bed bound. My husband (my rock) and I have been everywhere and tried everything.

To cut a long story short, it was suggested by a doctor in London that I should see an endocrinologist in Brussels. At that point I was on hydrocortisone, (blood pressure down to 80/30 which precipitated the prescription).

The endo always spent a lot of time lecturing us on diet. Lecturing is not too strong a word, he was very insistent that I should use coconut oil for cooking and not olive oil. Your book (*The Coconut Oil Miracle*) was shown to us along with a tub of oil. He was against the prevailing low-fat dogma, saying that fat is required by the body for making hormones.

The second strand of his diet theory was that I should eat a Paleolithic type diet: no grains, sugar, or dairy. Not too much fruit, loads of vegetables and salad, plus meat, fish, nuts, and seeds. My complaint was that I like yoghurt, so I was allowed two a week as a concession. This diet is very healthy especially when combined with the coconut oil and over time I recovered to a point where I decided to get off the meds. Since September 2004 I have been off all meds and my health since then has improved dramatically.

Apart from my recovered hormonal system (blood pressure now normal and stable) my energy is better, I sleep less but more refreshingly, I don't get night sweats almost nightly–I don't get them at all. I used to get a lot of leg pain, a sort of lactic acid feeling and that has dissipated in the past three to four months.

I think that my immune system is getting back to normal as I had the flu two months ago, was acutely ill and then recovered normally instead of languishing with fluey symptoms for months as previously. I have a few minor problems left, but I am hopeful that another six months should see me right.

My husband is also very healthy on this diet. He has lost 35 pounds (I lost 7 pounds, back to a normal weight of 125 pounds). Eighteen months ago just after turning 40 he took up squash again. As one of his friends commented, most people give up squash at 40, not take it up again!

I am very grateful to you for writing your book. I can safely say that it has changed our lives. We are members of the Weston A. Price Foundation, and I have reeducated myself on nutrition. Coconut oil along with a careful diet has restored health for both of us, and we enjoy cooking together as a hobby.

I love to hear how people are finding success. I would like to hear about your success too. Please write and share your experiences with me. You can reach me at:

Bruce Fife, ND
Coconut Research Center
P.O. Box 25203
Colorado Springs, CO 80936
E-mail: contact@coconutresearchcenter.org.

If you would like to learn more about the health benefits of coconut oil, visit my website at www.coconutresearchcenter.org. On this site you have the opportunity to sign up for a free subscription to my *Healthy Ways Newsletter*. This newsletter is sent out via e-mail every few weeks and gives the latest news on coconut research, diet, nutrition, and other health issues.

Seven-Day Whole Foods Challenge

Whole Foods Versus Processed Foods

The purpose of this challenge is to teach you how to identify, prepare, and eat healthy whole foods. If eating natural, whole foods is new to you, this challenge can be an invaluable teaching tool.

I recommend that all your foods be organically grown and processed. However, for this learning exercise we are not going to concern ourselves with this issue. We are just trying to learn what distinguishes natural, whole foods from overly processed or refined foods.

Whole foods are minimally processed. They are not chemically altered or extensively processed or refined. The term *whole foods* can be defined as any food you can catch, pick, grow, extract, or make at home using ordinary kitchen appliances. You can *catch* a fish, so it is a whole food. You cannot catch batter fried fish fillets. You can *pick* a cherry. You cannot pick a cherry toaster pastry. You can *grow* a grain of wheat. You cannot grow a chocolate chip cookie. You can *extract* milk from a cow and get whole milk. Cows do not produce skim milk. You can also extract sap from maple trees for maple syrup or honey from a honey comb. You cannot extract high fructose corn syrup from corn kernels or white sugar from sugar beets.

Any food you can make in your kitchen from *whole* ingredients can be considered a whole food. Homemade bread, muffins, and pancakes from whole wheat flour qualify. So does whole grain pasta. It can be made at home using a countertop pasta maker. Or you can buy whole grain pasta at the store (as long as it does not contain processed or chemical ingredients).

Fermented foods such as sauerkraut, pickles, yogurt, or cheese can be made at home and can be considered whole foods, as can dried foods such as fruit leather and raisins. Of course, you don't have to make all of these products at home. You can buy commercially available products; just make sure they are not refined and have no added chemicals or processed ingredients.

All fresh, raw fruits, vegetables, seeds, and nuts are whole foods. Fresh frozen foods would qualify too, as long as they don't have anything added. Although frozen vegetables have been blanched, the heat is only enough to retard enzymes and does not seriously affect the total nutrient content. They are not as good as fresh vegetables, but they are definitely better than canned. Read the ingredient labels on frozen foods, sometimes sugar and other ingredients are added.

If you purchase raw red meat, poultry, eggs, and fish, without any added ingredients, then they are whole foods. If the meat has been processed, smoked, dried, cured, or otherwise tampered with, then it is processed. This would include ham, bacon, bologna, pepperoni, pastrami, hot dogs, jerky, sausage, bratwurst, and such. It would also include any canned meats including tuna and chicken. Most processed meats contain many food additives. However, there are some meat packers who make "natural" processed meats. These are okay as long as the ingredients are truly natural. For example, you can eat sausage that is only ground pork and spices, without chemical preservatives or flavor enhancers.

Raw whole milk, cream, and cheeses are whole foods. Low-fat and fat-free milk, cheese, cottage cheese, and other dairy products are not. Look at ingredient labels. Some dairy products are made with powdered milk (definitely not a whole food) and other questionable ingredients.

Minimally processed oils are considered whole foods. Oils that are easily extracted from the source without the use of high temperatures, hydraulic presses, and chemical extracting agents would qualify. Virgin olive oil is a whole food. It is simply expelled from the olive fruit and filtered without further processing. Regular (non-virgin) olive oil is not a whole food, since it has gone though more processing and refining. Other whole oils include virgin coconut oil, red (virgin) palm oil, butter, and rendered animal fat. Grocery store vegetable oils, such as corn, soybean, canola, safflower, peanut, and sunflower oils, are not whole foods as they have undergone extensive processing. Shortening and margarine also are not whole foods.

Most all sugars and syrups are processed. All artificial sweeteners and sugar substitutes are processed. Brown sugar is not a natural sugar. It is white sugar with a little molasses added to it. Raw honey is a natural sweetener. Dehydrated sugarcane juice (Sucanat), dehydrated maple syrup, molasses, and dried fruit, like date sugar, are minimally processed. These "natural" sweeteners are usually grouped with whole foods, although their consumption should be limited because all sweeteners are low in nutrition and feed bacteria.

Herbs, spices, and salt generally fit into the whole foods category. Rock salt and sea salt are definitely whole foods and are good sources of trace minerals. Ordinary table salt is highly refined and usually has chemical additives. It is not a whole food.

Basically, anything that is cooked, altered chemically, or gone through a refining process and is sold in a can, plastic, box, or other type of sealed container is a processed food. If you can catch, pick, grow, or extract it, then chances are it's a whole food.

Now that you have an overview of what constitutes a whole food, it's time for a pop quiz. Take the following quiz to test your understanding of whole foods. The answers and a discussion follow. Try taking the test before looking at the answers.

Quiz
Which of the following would qualify as whole foods, and why?
1. Apple
2. Chicken nuggets
3. Pepperidge Farm Goldfish crackers
4. Tyson whole chicken
5. Pizza Hut pizza
6. Roman Meal whole grain bread

7. Minute Maid orange juice
8. Quaker Cinnamon Swirl instant oatmeal
9. Shredded wheat breakfast cereal
10. Granola bar
11. Frozen french fries
12. Egg Beaters
13. Cottage cheese
14. Peanut butter

Answers start on page 167.

Deceptive Advertising

You need to be cautious of marketing hype. In the grocery store, you will see foods labeled "All Natural Ingredients" or "Made with Whole Grains" and "Zero Trans Fats." These terms don't mean anything. They are just advertising ploys to fool you into thinking they are 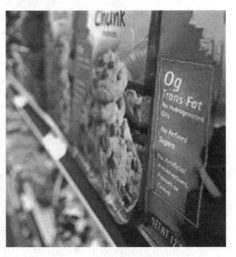 healthier than the competition. The term "All Natural Ingredients" is completely meaningless. If the ingredients in the food originally came from something natural, no matter how much refining and processing they have gone through, and no matter what other "non-natural" chemicals have been added to it, manufacturers can make that claim.

continued on next page

Nutrition Facts	
Serving Size 1 cup (228g)	
Servings Per Container 2	

Amount Per Serving	
Calories 260	Calories from Fat 120

	% Daily Value*
Total Fat 13g	20%
Saturated Fat 5g	25%
Trans Fat 2g	
Cholesterol 30mg	10%
Sodium 660mg	28%
Total Carbohydrate 31g	10%
Dietary Fiber 0g	0%
Sugars 5g	
Protein 5g	

Vitamin A 4%	•	Vitamin C 2%	
Calcium 15%	•	Iron 4%	

*Percent Daily Values are based on a 2,000 calorie diet. Your Daily Values may be higher or lower depending on your calorie needs:

	Calories:	2,000	2,500
Total Fat	Less than	65g	80g
Sat Fat	Less than	20g	25g
Cholesterol	Less than	300mg	300mg
Sodium	Less than	2,400mg	2,400mg
Total Carbohydrate		300g	375g
Dietary Fiber		25g	30g
Calories per gram:			
Fat 9	•	Carbohydrate 4	• Protein 4

The term "Made with Whole Grain" is also meaningless. Look at the ingredient label. Usually the first item is enriched wheat flour. This is another way of saying "processed white flour." Whole wheat flour does not need to be enriched with vitamins and minerals, but white flour does. In processing whole wheat into white flour, many vitamins and minerals are removed. In the past, this has led to widespread nutritional deficiencies. Therefore, by law manufacturers are required to add back a few (but not all) of the essential nutrients that have been removed. The term "wheat flour" on an ingredient label is a gimmick to trick customers into thinking the product is made from whole wheat. "Wheat flour" usually means "white flour" made from wheat. You want a product made with 100 percent *whole* wheat. When products advertise an item as being made with "whole grains" it often means that whole wheat or some other whole grain has been added, but that is not necessarily the main ingredient.

The term "Zero Trans Fats" is another lie. Manufacturers can legally make this claim if a serving contains less than half a gram of trans fats. Therefore, in a package of "Zero Trans Fat" cookies, for example, one serving could be equal to one cookie. This cookie can have nearly .5 grams of trans fats. How many people will only eat one cookie? Essentially none! So, you end up eating four or five cookies or, if you're really hungry, maybe 10. You add up all the trans fats and you're eating a lot! How do you tell if something really is trans fat free? Look at the ingredient label. If it lists partially hydrogenated vegetable oil, margarine, or shortening, then it contains trans fats. Don't eat it. ■

Answers

1. Yes. This was an easy one. A fresh raw apple is a whole food. Dried apple slices would be as well as long as they do not have added preservatives or sugar.
2. No. Chickens don't have nuggets. These bite-size chicken pieces are highly processed. They are made from meat that has been stripped off the bones. Often, the dark meat is bleached to make it appear white. Both dark and white meat are mixed together and shaped into nuggets and covered in a breaded coating. Flavor enhancers such as MSG are added.
3. No. Pepperidge Farm may call them "goldfish," but I promise you that there are no cheddar flavored fish swimming around in the wild.
4. Yes. A whole, uncooked chicken is a whole food.
5. No. Restaurant and frozen pizzas are not whole foods. They are made with white flour and the toppings contain highly processed meats, cheeses, and other ingredients.
6. No. Although bread may say it contains whole grain or whole wheat, they often contain just as much or more white enriched wheat along with high fructose corn syrup, soybean oil, preservatives, and an assortment of other additives.
7. No. Prepared orange juice is processed. It is pasteurized and often condensed. And may have added sugar, even if it does not list sugar on the label. Manufacturers are allowed to add enough sugar to meet certain limits without listing the added sugar on the ingredient label.
8. No. Instant oatmeal is processed so that it cooks within three minutes or less. It also contains sugar, artificial sweeteners, artificial flavorings, and other additives. "Old Fashion" oats, however, are considered a whole food. Nothing is added or removed from the edible portion of the grain.
9. No. All cold cereals are highly processed, and most contain preservatives, sugar, and other additives.
10. No. A granola bar may sound healthy, but these "health" bars are not much more than glorified candy bars loaded with sugars and other questionable ingredients.

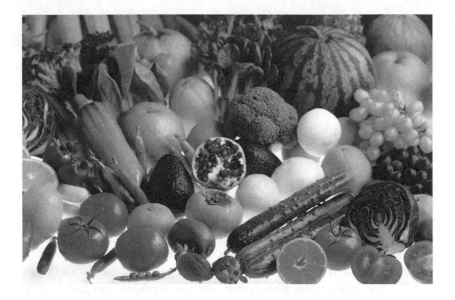

11. No. Although they look like only cut potatoes, they are usually precooked and contain hydrogenated or other questionable oils.
12. No. Egg Beaters is definitely not a whole food. Chickens do not lay yolkless eggs. Egg Beaters are egg whites without the yolk. It's a joke.
13. Yes. If it is full fat. Low fat dairy, however, is not since it is manipulated to remove the natural milkfat.
14. Depends. Peanuts are a whole food. Ground peanuts? Also a whole food. Ground peanuts with a little salt? Still a whole food. Skippy peanut butter? Nope. Read the label. The second ingredient in Skippy peanut butter is sugar. It also contains hydrogenated vegetable oil. It is junk food disguised as a healthy choice.

Just because many of your favorite foods may be on the Arthritis Forming Diet list doesn't mean you can't ever enjoy them again. On the contrary, many of these foods can be eaten freely, *if,* and this is a big if, you make them yourself using whole ingredients. For instance, you can enjoy pizza, but make the crust using whole wheat flour and wholesome toppings. The same with hamburgers and french fries.

French fries? Yes, you can eat fried potatoes, if they are made from fresh potatoes and cooked in a healthy fat such as coconut or palm oil. When making hamburgers, use fresh ground beef and whole wheat buns. You can even enjoy an occasional dessert if you make it with natural ingredients. Cakes and cookies can be made with whole grains and can taste just as good as if they were made with white flour. Although I don't recommend you eat desserts every day, they can be consumed on occasion.

The Seven-Day Challenge: The Rules

In this challenge, you earn points from the types of foods you eat. At the end of seven days, all of your points will be tallied. You get one point for each whole food that you eat, and you lose one point for each refined food that you eat.

Food mixtures (soup, stir-fry, salad) that contain only whole ingredients are whole foods. Whole foods and whole food mixes contain *only* whole ingredients. If mixed foods have *any* processed ingredients, they count as processed food. Some examples: baked chicken coated in *white flour*; fish fried in *soybean oil*; baked apple with *sugar* topping; anything with partially hydrogenated vegetable oil, high fructose corn syrup, MSG, artificial flavors or colors, preservatives, or any chemical additives. For this exercise, water is a zero food. You neither gain points nor lose them, so you can drink water as you like.

The point system is based on serving size. Serving size varies depending on the type of food. One serving equals 1 point (or -1 point, as the case may be). For this exercise you will use the following guidelines to estimate serving size. These are not necessarily standard serving sizes used in the food industry, but a simplified system to make calculating the points as easy as possible for our exercise:

Grains and cereal: 1 cup
Beverages: 1 cup
Medium-sized fruit (apple): 1 whole
Small-sized fruit (blueberries): ½ cup
Large-sized fruit (melon): 1 cup, sliced
Medium-sized vegetable (carrot): 1 whole

169

Small-sized vegetable (peas): ½ cup
Large-sized vegetable (eggplant): ½ cup, chopped
Bread: 1 slice
Buns and rolls (hamburger): ½ piece, top or bottom
Meat and fish: 3 ounces, about the size of a deck of playing cards
Mixed foods (soup, casserole): 1 cup
Snack foods (chips, pretzels, popcorn): ½ cup

Round up any portion that does not equal a full serving. For example, if you eat half an apple, count it as 1 serving. If you eat 1½ cups of soup, round up to 2 servings; ¾ cup of soup counts as 1 serving.

Let's look at a few examples:

A baked potato = 1 point
A baked potato with margarine = -1
A baked potato with butter = 1
Mashed potatoes from a box = -1
Mashed potatoes from real potatoes = 1
Whole oats, cooked = 1
Instant oatmeal = -1
Whole oats with 1% milk = -1
Whole oats with whole milk and honey = 1
Raw carrot = 1
Cooked carrot = 1
Sugar glazed carrots = -1
Grilled chicken breast = 1
Chicken nuggets = -1
Canned peas = -1
Homemade soup = 1
Canned soup = -1
Broccoli sautéed in virgin coconut oil = 1
Egg fried in corn oil = -1
A slice of whole wheat bread with butter = 1
A slice of whole wheat bread and jam = -1

Got the idea? Now let's talk about food combinations. The best way to do this is to look at an example: a turkey sandwich with two slices of white bread, 1 tablespoon of mayonnaise, two slices of tomato, one lettuce leaf, and 2 ounces of turkey lunchmeat. This exercise would become too cumbersome if we tried to count each individual item of food and attempted to figure out a serving size for each. It is much easier to take the entire sandwich as a whole. First, we need to decide if the sandwich would qualify as a whole food or not. Since it contains white bread and turkey lunchmeat, it clearly would not. Next, you need to estimate the serving size. Two slices of bread constitutes two servings, giving you -2 points. None of the fillings in the sandwich equals a full serving individually, so count them all as one mixed food. Since one ingredient in the filling is processed (lunchmeat) the entire filling is given -1 point. The sandwich earns a total of -3 points.

If the sandwich was made with whole wheat bread and the turkey lunchmeat, the total would come to 1, (2 for each slice of whole wheat bread and -1 for the lunchmeat). If the turkey lunchmeat was replaced with real sliced turkey, the total would come to 3. If you add a serving of potato chips (-1), the total drops to 2.

Now, let's say you go to the food court at the mall and order a plate of chicken chow mein. First of all, *what are you doing???* Fast foods, and in fact most restaurant foods, are almost always made with processed ingredients. Well, it happens to the best of us sometimes. Okay, you could try to figure out everything in the dish, the chicken, mushrooms, bean sprouts, noodles, etc. plus the side dish of rice and figure serving sizes of each. But this would become too cumbersome. Treat it as a mixed dish and calculate the side dish of rice separately. Estimate the serving size of the chicken-vegetable mixture. Let's say 1½ cups. We will round that up to 2 cups for a total of -2 points. Although you may see mostly chicken and vegetables in the dish, there are many hidden ingredients such as soybean oil, high fructose corn syrup, MSG, cornstarch, etc. This is a processed food, therefore, the reason for the -2 points.

Next, we need to account for the side dish of rice. The rice served in restaurants is almost always *white* rice—a processed grain. Fried rice is also made with white rice. Be very careful about portions. A

171

serving of rice, according to our rules, is 1 cup. If you eat the 1½ cups of rice, which is about what the average Chinese restaurant sets before you, then that's -2 points. Total for the meal is -4 points.

What if you decide against the chicken chow mein and instead order four McDonald's Chicken McNuggets and a small fries? Count all the McNuggets as one serving and the fries as one serving (-2 total). If you eat the four McNuggets and then decide to go back and get more, that's two servings. And don't pretend that a supersized order of fries is a single serving, count it as -2.

Most restaurant portions are *huge*. Just because the Cheesecake Factory serves you a one pound slice of cheesecake or two pounds of pasta on a platter-sized plate doesn't mean that it is one serving! You add or subtract points per serving.

Got the picture? Obviously, there is a lot of room for fudging, particularly with portion sizes, as these will usually be estimates. That's okay. This is not a science experiment. It's an exercise—a learning aid—to help you think about the foods you eat and to encourage you to make healthier dietary choices. This system obviously isn't perfect, but it is an excellent teaching tool for those who are just learning about the difference between processed and whole foods.

When scoring, be totally honest. This exercise is to help you. You aren't competing with anyone. You want an honest account. If you get a low score or even a negative one, view it as informative. Learn from it and use it to help yourself improve.

Record your number of points for each meal and each snack and keep a daily tally. At the end of seven days, count your total points. Compare your total to the scores below.

Seven-Day Challenge Score

- 60 or more points: Excellent. You are on your way to better health.
- 20-59 points: Good. You are learning how to make good choices.
- 10-19 points: Improvement needed. Continue to work on your food choices.
- 0-10 points: Trouble is just waiting to happen.
- -1 or fewer points: Call the ambulance! Need I say more?

How did you do? Are you on track? If not, keep working on it. For most people, converting over to a whole foods diet is a challenge. You don't need to do it overnight. You can make the change gradually and get accustomed to the new way of eating. In time, you will make it a habit.

The purpose of the above exercise is to teach you about whole foods and about making wise food choices. It is not, however, exactly the same as the Anti-Arthritis Diet recommended in Chapter 7. Although this is a good diet for those suffering from arthritis, the *low-carb whole foods diet* goes a step further. With the low-carb whole foods diet you eat whole foods as described here, but you limit the high carbohydrate foods such as grains, natural sweeteners, fruits, and starchy vegetables.

High carb foods, even if they are whole foods, can feed unfriendly bacteria in the mouth and gut. Reducing the amount of these foods in your diet will be beneficial in your battle to conquer arthritis. Once you have achieved the results you desire, you can increase your carbohydrate consumption.

Whole Foods ∾ Processed Foods

Whole foods are those you can catch, pick, grow, extract, or make at home using ordinary kitchen appliances. Any food that is cooked, altered chemically, or has gone through a refining process and is sold in a can, plastic, box, or other type of sealed container is a processed food.

References

Chapter 2: The Many Faces of Arthritis

1. Swedberg, J.A. and Steinbauer, J.R. Osteoarthritis. *American Family Physician* 1992;45(2):557-568.

2. Head, J. Osteoarthritis in its relation to mouth infection. *Journal of Bone and Joint Surgery* 1915;S2-13:71-85.

3. Ramiro, I., et al. Proliferative osteoarthritis and osteoarthrosis in 15 snakes. *Journal of Zoo and Wildlife Medicine* 2000;31:20-27.

4. Kramer, H.M. and Curhan, G. The association between gout and nephrolithiasis: The National Health and Nutrition Examination Survey III, 1988–1994. *Am J of Kid Dis* 2002;40:37–42.

5. Kramer, J.H., et al. The association between gout and nephrolithiasis in men: The Health Professionals' Follow-up Study. *Kidney International* 2003;64:1022–1026.

6. Ebringer, A. The cross-tolerance hypothesis. HLA-B27 and ankylosing spondylitis. *Br J Rheumatol* 1983;22(suppl 2):53-66.

7. Geczy, A.F., et al. HLA-B27, Klebsiella and ankylosing spondylitis: biological and chemical studies *Immunol Rev* 1983;70:23-50.

8. Aho, K., et al. HL-A27 in reactive arthritis following infection. *Ann Rheum Dis* 1975;34:29-30.

9. Ebringer, R.W., et al. Sequential studies in ankylosing spondylitis: association of *Klebsiella pneumoniae* and active disease. *Ann Rheum Dis* 1978;37:146-151.

10. Nuki, G. Ankylosing spondylitis, HLA B27 and beyond. *Lancet* 1998;351:767-769.

11. Hakansson, U., et al. HLA antigen B27 in cases of joint affections in an outbreak of salmonellosis. *Scand J Infect Dis* 1976;8:245-248.

12. Ablin, J.N., et al. Fibromyalgia, infection and vaccination: two more parts in the etiological puzzle. *J Autoimmun* 2006;27:145-152.

13. Buskila, D., et al. Etiology of fibromyalgia: the possible role of infection and vaccination. *Autoimmun Rev* 2008;8:41-43.

Chapter 3: What Causes Arthritis?

1. Brooks, P.M., et al. NSAID and osteoarthritis—help or hindrance. *J Rheumatol* 1982;9:3-5.

2. Newman, N.M. and Ling, R.S.M.. Acetabular bone destruction related to non-steroidal anti-inflammatory drugs. *Lancet* 1985;ii;11-13.

3. Moseley, J.B., et al. A controlled trial of arthroscopic surgery for osteoarthritis of the knee. *New England Journal of Medicine* 2002;347:81-88.

4. Volpe, A., et al. Chikungunya arthritis: report of 6 cases. *Reumatismo* 2008;60:136-140.

5. Kessel, S. and Wittenberg, C.E. Joint infection in a young patient caused by Streptococcus uberis, a pathogen of bovine mastitis—a case report. *Z Othop Unfall* 2008;146:507-509.

6. de Almeida, A.E., et al. Septic arthritis due to Haemophilus influenzae serotype a in the post-vaccination era in Brazil. *J Med Microbiol* 2008; 57:1311-1312.

7. Kathresal, A., et al. A rare case of Candida arthritis in a hemodialysis patient. *Am J Med Sci* 2008;336:437-440.

8. Moser, C., et al. Infective arthritis: bacterial 23S rRNA gene sequencing as a supplementary diagnostic method. *Open Microbiol J* 2008;2:85-88.

9. Fe Marques, A., et al. Septic arthritis of the knee due to Prevotella loescheii following tooth extraction. *Med Oral Patol Oral Cir Bucal* 2008;13:E505-E507.

10. Vera, M. Jr., et al. Antimicrobial prophylaxis in oral surgery and dental procedures. *Med Oral Patol Oral Cir Bucal* 2007;12:E44-E52.

11. Fitzgerald, R.H., et al. Anaerobic septic arthritis. *Clin Orthop Relat Res* 1982;164:141-148.

12. Nolla, J.M., et al. Pyarthrosis in patients with rheumatoid arthritis: a detailed analysis of 10 cases and literature review. *Semin Arthritis Rheum* 2000;30:121-126.

13. Aderinto, J., et al. Early syphilis: a cause of mono-arthritis of the knee. *Ann R Coll Surg Engl* 2008;90:W1-W3.

14. Rojo, C.W., et al. Prevalence and cervical human papilloma virus associated factors in patients with rheumatoid arthritis. *Ginecol Obstet Mex* 2008;76:9-17.

15. Rohekar, S., et al. Symptomatic acute reactive arthritis after an outbreak of salmonella. *J Rheumatol* 2008;35:1599-1602.

16. Vaahtovuo, J., et al. Fecal microbiota in early rheumatoid arthritis. *J Rheumatol* 2008;35:1477-1479.

17. Sipahi, O.R., et al. Streptococcus equismillis associated septic arthritis/ prosthetic joint infection. *Mikrobiyol Bul* 2008;42:515-518.

18. Cole, B.C. and Griffiths, M.M. Triggering and exacerbating of autoimmune arthritis by the Mycoplasma arthritidis superantigen MAM. *Arthritis and Rheumatism* 1993;36:994-1002.

19. Senior, B.W., et al. Evidence that patients with rheumatoid arthritis have asymptomatic 'non-significant' Proteus mirabilis bacteriuria more frequently than healthy controls. *J Infect* 1999;38:99-106.

20. Senior, B.W., et al. Evidence that patients with rheumatoid arthritis have asymptomatic 'non-significant' Proteus mirabilis bacteriuria more frequently than healthy controls. *J Infect* 1999;38:99-106.

21. Ebringer, A. and Rashid, T. Rheumatoid arthritis is an autoimmune disease triggered by Proteus urinary tract infection. *Clin Dev Immunol* 2006;13:41-48.

22. Toivanen, A. Alphaviruses: an emerging cause of arthritis? *Curr Opin Rheumatol* 2008;20:486-490.

23. Kobayashi, S., et al. Molecular aspects of rheumatoid arthritis: role of environmental factors. *FEBS J* 2008;275:4456-4462.

24. Bokarewa, M., et al. Arthritogenic dsRNA is present in synovial fluid from rheumatoid arthritis patients with an erosive disease course. *Eur J Immunol* 2008;38:3237-3244.

25. Amital, H., et al. Role of infectious agents in systemic rheumatic diseases. *Clin Exp Rheumatol* 2008;26:S27-S32.

26. Kozireva, S.V., et al. Incidence and clinical significance of parvovirus B19 infection in patients with rheumatoid arthritis. *J Rheumatol* 2008;35:1265-1270.

27. Rashid, T. and Ebringer, A. Ankylosing spondylitis is linked to Klebsiella— the evidence. *Clin Rheumatol* 2007;26:858-864.

28. Amanai, T., et al. Micro-CT analysis of experimental Candida osteoarthritis in rats. *Mycopathologia* 2008;166:133-141.

29. Yagupsky, P. Trimethoprim-sulfamethoxazole for osteoarthritis caused by Staphylococcus aureus or Kingella kingae. *Pediatr Infect Dis J* 2008;27:1042-1043.

30. Luna-Pizarro, D., et al. Monoarthritis of the knee with unusual lesions in adults associated with varicella-zoster virus infection. *Arthroscopy* 2009;25:106-108.

31. Rozin, A. Is osteoarthritis an infection-associated disease and a target for chemotherapy? *Chemotherapy* 2007;53:1-9.

32. Mahilton, M.e. et al. Simultaneous gout and pyarthrosis. *Arch Intern Med* 1980;140:9170919.

33. O'Connell, P.G., et al. Coexistent gout and septic arthritis: a report of two cases and literature review. *Clin Exp Rheumatol* 1985;3:265-267.

34. Edwards, G.S. Jr and Russell, I.J. Pneumococcal arthritis complicating gout. Case report and literature review. *J Rheumatol* 1980;7:907-910.

35. Benjamin, C.M., et al. Joint and limb symptoms in children after immunisation with measles, mumps, and rubella vaccine. *British Medical Journal* 1992;304:1075-1078.

36. Mitchell, L.A., et al. Chronic rubella vaccine-associated arthropathy. *Archives of Internal Medicine* 1993;153:2268-2274.

37. Nussinovitch, M., et al Arthritis after mumps and measles vaccination. *Arch Dis Child* 1995;72:348-349.

38. Ogra, P.L., et al. Rubella-virus infection in juvenile rheumatoid arthritis. *Lancet* 1975;24:1157-1161.

39. Pattison, E., et al. Environmental risk factors for the development of psoriatic arthritis: results from a case-control study. *Ann Rheum Dis* 2008;67:672-676.

40. Geier, D.A. and Geier, M.R. Rubella vaccine and arthritic adverse reactions: an analysis of the Vaccine Adverse Events Reporting System (VAERS) database from 1991 through 1998. *Clin Exp Rheumatol* 2001;19:724-726.

41. Mitchell, L.A., et al. Rubella virus vaccine associated arthropathy in postpartum immunized women: influence of preimmunization serologic status on development of joint manifestations. *J Rheumatol* 2000;27:418-423.

42. Valenzuela-Suarez, H., et al. A seventy-four-year-old man with bilateral conjunctival hyperemia, urinary symptoms, and secondary reactive arthritis following the administration of the BCG vaccine. *Gac Med Mex* 2008;144:345-347.

43. de Almeida, A.E., et al. Septic arthritis due to Haemophilus influenzae serotype a in the post-vaccination era in Brazil. *J Med Microbiol* 2008;57:1311-1312.

44. Dudelzak, J., et al. New-onset psoriasis and psoriatic arthritis in a patient treated with Bacillus Calmette-Guerin (BCG) immunotherapy. *J Drugs Dermatol* 2008;7:684.

45. Tinazzi, E., et al. Reactive arthritis following BCG immunotherapy for bladder carcinoma. *Clin Rheumatol* 2005;24:425-427.

46. Garyfallou, G.T. Mycobacterial sepsis following intravesical instillation of bacillus Calmette-Guerin. *Acad Emerg Med* 1996;3:157-160.

47. Hirayama, T., et al. Anaphylactoid purpura after intravesical therapy using bacillus Calmette-Guerin for superficial bladder cancer. *Hinyokika Kiyo* 2008;54:127-129.

48. Bruce, M.G., et al. Epidemiology of Haemophilus influenzae serotypea, North American Artic, 2000-2005. *Emerg Infect Dis* 2008;14:48-55.

49. Thoon, K.C., et al. Epidemiology of invasive Haemophilus influenzae type b disease in Singapore children, 1994-2003. *Vaccine* 2007;25:6482-6489.

50. Schattner, A. Consequence or coincidence? The occurrence, pathogenesis and significance of autoimmune manifestations after viral vaccines. *Vaccine* 2005;23:3876-3886.

51. Shoenfeld, Y. and Aron-Maor, A. Vaccination and autoimmunity-'vaccinosis': a dangerous liaison? *J Autoimmun* 2000;14:1-10.

52. Paterson, D.L. and Patel, A. Bacillus Calmette-Guerin (BCG) immunotherapy for bladder cancer: review of complications and their treatment. *Aust N Z J Surg* 1998;68:340-344.

53. Gluck, T. and Muller-Ladner, U. Vaccination in patients with chronic rheumatic or autoimmune diseases. *Clin Infect Dis* 2008;46:1459-1465.

54. Amanai, T., et al. Micro-CT analysis of experimental Candida osteoarthritis in rats. *Mycopathologia* 2008;166:133-141.

55. Kathresal, A. A rare case of Candida arthritis in a hemodialysis patient. *Am J Med Sci* 2008;336:437-440.

56. Choi, B.K., et al. Diversity of cultivable and uncultivable oral spirochetes from a patient with severe destructive periodontitis. *Infection and Immunity* 1994;62:1889-1895.

57. Matsuzaki, K. Molecular action mechanisms and membrane recognition of membrane-acting antimicrobial peptides. *Yakugaku Zasshi* 1997;117:253-264.

58. Kondo, E. and Kanai, K. Bactericidal activity of the membrane fraction isolated from phagocytes of mice and its stimulation by melittin. *Jpn J Med Sci Biol* 1986;39:9-20.

59. Stocker, J.F. and Traynor, J.R. The action of various venoms on Escherichia coli. *J Appl Bacteriol* 1986;61:383-388.

60. Perumal Samy, R., et al. In vitro antimicrobial activity of natural toxins and animal venoms tested against Burkholderia pseudomallei. *BMC Infect Dis* 2006;6:100.

61. Lubke, L.L. and Garon, C.F. The antimicrobial agent melittin exhibits powerful in vitro inhibitory effects on the Lyme diseases spirochete. *Clin Infect Dis* 1997;25:S48-51.

62. Boutrin, M.C., et al. The effects of bee (Apis meliifera) venom phospholipase A2 on Trypanosoma brucei brucei and enterobacteria. *Exp Parasitol* 2008;119:246-251.

63. Esser, A.F., et al. Disassembly of viral membranes by complement independent of channel formation. *Proc Natl Acad Sci USA* 1979;76:5843-5847.

64. Yasin, B., et al. Evaluation of the inactivation of infectious Herpes simplex virus by host-defense peptides. *Eur J Clin Microbiol Infect Dis* 2000;19:187-194.

65. Fenard, D., et al. Secreted phospholipases A(2), a new class of HIV inhibitors that block virus entry into host cells. *J Clin Invest* 1999;104:611-618.

66. Deregnaucourt, C. and Schrevel, J. Bee venom phospholipase A2 induces stage-specific growth arrest of the intraerythrocytic *Plasmodium falciparum* via modifications of human serum components. *J Biol Chem* 2000;275:39973-39980.

67. Boman, H.G., et al. Antibacterial and antimalarial properties of peptides that are cecropin-melittin hybrids. *FEBS Lett* 1989;259:103-106.

68. Choi, S.H. and Kang, S.S. Therapeutic effect of bee venom in sows with hypogalactia syndrome postpartum. *J Vet Sci* 2001;2:121-124.

69. Choi, S.H., et al. Effect of apitherapy in piglets with preweaning diarrhea. *Am J Clin Med* 2003;31:321-326.
70. Kang, S.S. et al. The effect of whole bee venom on arthritis. *Am J Chin Med* 2002;30:73-80.
71. Lee, J.Y., et al. Inhibitory effect of whole bee venom in adjuvant-induced arthritis. *In Vivo* 2005;19:801-805.
72. Luo, H. et al. Effect of bee venom on adjuvant induced arthritis in rats. *Zhong Nan Da Xue Xue Bao Yi Xue Ban* 2006;31:948-951.
73. Liu, X.D., et al. Clinical randomized study of bee-sting therapy for rheumatoid arthritis. *Zhen Ci Yan Jiu* 2008;33:197-200.
74. Lee, J.D., et al. An overview of bee venom acupuncture in the treatment of arthritis. *Evid Based Complement Alternat Med* 2005;2:79-84.
75. Kwon, G.R. Clinical study on treatment of rheumatoid arthritis by bee venom therapy. *Proc Congress Kor Med* 1998;130-131.
76. Wang, O.H., et al. Clinical study on effectiveness of bee venom therapy on degenerative knee arthritis. *J Kor Acu Max Soc* 2001;18:35-47.
77. Businco, L., et al. Disseminated arthritis and osteitis by Candida albicans in a two month old infant receiving parenteral nutrition. *Acta Paediatr Scand* 1977;66:393-395.
78. Lossos, I.S., et al. Septic arthritis of the glenohumeral joint. A report of 11 cases and review of the literature. *Medicine (Baltimore)* 1998;77:177-187.

Chapter 4: The Tooth Connection

1. Price, W.A. *Dental Infections, Volume II*. La Mesa, CA:Price-Pottenger Nutrition Foundation, 1923.
2. Cecil, R.L. The bacteriology of dental infections and its relation to systemic disease. *New York State Journal of Medicine* 1932;32:1242-1245.
3. Billings, F. Chronic focal infections and their etiologic relations to arthritis and nephritis. *Archives of Internal Medicine* 1912;9:484-453.
4. Price, W.A. *Dental Infections, Volumes I and II*. La Mesa, CA:Price-Pottenger Nutrition Foundation, 1923.
5. Price, W.A. *Dental Infections, Volume I*. La Mesa, CA:Price-Pottenger Nutrition Foundation, 1923.
6. Miluls, T.R., et al. Antibody responses to Porphyromonas gingivalis (P. gingivalis) in subjects with rheumatoid arthritis and periodontitis. *Int Immunopharmacol* 2009;9:38-42.
7. Moen, K., et al. Synovial inflammation in active rheumatoid arthritis and psoriatic arthritis facilitates trapping of a variety of oral bacterial DNAs. *Clin Exp Rheumatol* 2006;24:656-663.
8. Sonsale, P.D., et al. Arthritis of the knee due to Fusobacterium necrophorum. *J Clin Microbiol* 2004;42:3369-3370.

9. Flesher, S.A. and Bottone, E.J. Eikenella corrodens cellulites and arthritis of the knee. *J Clin Microbiol* 1989;27:2606-2608.

10. Steingruber, I. et al. Infection of a total hip arthroplasty with Prevotella loeschii. *Clin Orthop Relat Res* 2004;418:222-224.

11. Pischon, N., et al. Association among rheumatoid arthritis, oral hygiene, and periodontitis. *J Periodontol* 2008;79:979-986.

12. de Pablo, P., et al. Association of periodontal disease and tooth loss with rheumatoid arthritis in the US population. *J Rheumatol* 2008;35:70-76.

13. Kasser, U.R., et al. Risk for periodontal disease in patients with longstanding rheumatoid arthritis. *Arthritis Rheum* 1997;40:2248-2251.

14. Nilsson, M. and Kopp, S. Gingivitis and periodontitis are related to repeated high levels of circulating tumor necrosis factor-alpha in patients with rheumatoid arthritis. *J Periodontal* 2008;79:1689-1696.

15. Ogrendik, M. Periodontopathic bacteria and rheumatoid arthritis: is there a link? *J Clin Rheumatol* 2008;14:310-311.

16. Pers, J.O., et al. Anti-TNF-alpha immunotherapy is associated with increased gingival inflammation without clinical attachment loss in subjects with rheumatoid arthritis. *J Periodontol* 2008;79:1645-1651.

17. Thé, J. and Ebersole, J.L. Rheumatoid factor (RF) distribution in periodontal disease. *J Clin Immunol* 1991;11:132-142.

18. Mercado, F.B., et al Relationship between rheumatoid arthritis and periodontitis. *J Periodontal* 2001;72:779-787.

19. Havemose-Poulsen, A., et al. Periodontal and hematological characteristics associated with aggressive periodontitis, juvenile idiopathic arthritis, and rheumatoid arthritis. *J Periodontol* 2006;77:280-288.

20. Bartold, P.M., et al Periodontitis and rheumatoid arthritis: a review. *J Periodontal* 2005;76:2066-2074.

21. Rosenstein, E.D., et al. Hypothesis: the humoral immune response to oral bacteria provides a stimulus for the development of rheumatoid arthritis. *Inflammation* 2004;28:311-318.

22. Ramamurthy, N.S., et al. Experimental arthritis in rats induces biomarkers of periodontitis which are ameliorated by gene therapy with tissue inhibitor of matrix metalloproteinases. *J Periodontol* 2005;76:229-233.

23. Ogrendik, M., et al Serum antibodies to oral anaerobic bacteria in patients with rheumatoid arthritis. *MedGenMed* 2005;7:2-11.

24. de Pablo, P., et al. Association of periodontal disease and tooth loss with rheumatoid arthritis in the US population. *J Rheumatol* 2008;35:70-76.

25. Bartold, P.M., et al. Periodontitis and rheumatoid arthritis; a review. *J Periodontiol* 2005;76:2066-2074.

26. Al-Katma, M.K., et al. Control of periodontal infection reduces the severity of active rheumatoid arthritis. *J Clin Rheumatol* 2007;13:134-137.

27. Endresen, G.K. Mycoplasma blood infection in chronic fatigue and fibromyalgia syndromes. *Rheumatol Int* 2003;23:211-215.
28. Lindqvist, C. and Slatis, P. Dental bacteremia—a neglected cause of arthroplasty infections? Three hip cases. *Acta Orthop Scan* 1985;56:506-508.
29. Waldman, B.J., et al. Total knee arthroplasty infections associated with dental procedures. *Clin Orthop Relat Res* 1997;343:164-172.
30. Kingston, R., et al Antibiotic prophylaxis for dental or urological procedures following hip or knee replacement. *J Infect* 2002;45:243-245.

Chapter 5: The Root of the Problem

1. Meinnig, G.E. *Root Canal Cover-Up*. La Mesa, CA:Price-Pottenger Nutrition Foundation, 1994.
2. Fardy, C.H., et al. Toxic shock syndrome secondary to a dental abscess. *International Journal of Oral and Maxillofacial Surgery*.1999;28:60-61.
3. Price, W.A. *Dental Infections, Volume I*. La Mesa, CA:Price-Pottenger Nutrition Foundation, 1923.
4. Ebringer, A. and Rashid, T. Rheumatoid arthritis is an autoimmune disease triggered by Proteus urinary tract infection. *Clin Dev Immunol* 2006;13:41-48.
5. Amith, H.V., et al. Effect of oil pulling on plaque and gingivitis. *JOHCD* 2007;1:12-18.

Chapter 6: Nature's Antibiotic

1. Isaacs, C.E. and Thormar, H. The role of milk-derived antimicrobial lipids as antiviral and antibacterial agents, in *Immunology of Milk and the Neonate* (Mestecky, J., et al., eds) 1991, Plenum Press.
2. Isaacs, C.E. and Thormar, H. The role of milk-derived antimicrobial lipids as antiviral and antibacterial agents. *Adv Exp Med Biol* 1991;310:159-165.
3. Isaacs, C.E., et al. Antiviral and antibacterial lipids in human milk and infant formula feeds. *Arch Dis Child* 1990;65:861-864.
4. Bergsson, G., et al. In vitro inactivation of Chlamydia trachomatis by fatty acids and monoglycerides. *Antimicrobial Agents and Chemotherapy* 1998;42:2290-2292.
5. Petschow, B.W., et al Susceptibility of Helicobacter pylori to bactericidal properties of medium-chain monoglycerides and free fatty acids. *Antimicrobial Agents and Chemotherapy* 1996;40;302-306.
6. Holland, K.T., et al. The effect of glycerol monolaurate on growth of, and production of toxic shock syndrome toxin-1 and lipase by, Staphylococcus aureus. *Journal of Antimicrobial Chemotherapy* 1994;33:41-55.
7. Sun, C.Q., et al. Antibacterial actions of fatty acids and monoglycerides against Helicobacter pylori. *FEMS Immunol Med Microbiol* 2003;36:9-17.

8.Bergsson, G., et al. Killing of Gram-positive cocci by fatty acids and monoglycerides. *APMIS* 2001;109:670-678.

9. Bergsson, G., et al. In vitro susceptibilities of Neisseria gonorrhoeae to fatty acids and monoglycerides. *Antimicrob Agents Chemother* 1999;43:2790-2792.

10. Ogbolu, D.O., et al, In vitro antimicrobial properties of coconut oil on Candida species in Ibadan, Nigeria. *J Med Food* 2007;10:384-387.

11. Bergsson, G., et al. In vitro killing of Candida albicans by fatty acids and monoglycerides. *Antimicrob Agents Chemother* 2001;45:3209-3212.

12. Chadeganipour, M, and Haims, A. Antifungal activities of pelargonic and capric acid on Miscrosporum gypseum. *Mycoses* 2001;44:109-112.

13. Isaacs, E.E., et al. Inactivation of enveloped viruses in human bodily fluids by purified lipid. *Annals of the New York Academy of Sciences* 1994;724:465-471.

14. Bartolotta, S., et al. Effect of fatty acids on arenavirus replication: inhibition of virus production by lauric acid. *Arch Virol* 2001;146:777-790.

15. Thormar, H., et al. Inactivation of visna virus and other enveloped viruses by free fatty acids and monoglycerides. *Ann NY Acad Sci* 1994;724:465-471.

16. Hornung, B., et al. Lauric acid inhibits the maturation of vesicular stomatitis virus. *J Gen Virol* 1994;75:353-361.

17. Thormar, H., et al. Inactivation of enveloped viruses and killing of cells by fatty acids and monoglycerides. *Antimicrob Agents Chemother* 1987;31:27-31.

18. Vazquez, C., et al. Eucaloric substitution of medium chain triglycerides for dietary long chain fatty acids improves body composition and lipid profile in a patient with human immunodeficiency virus lipodystrophy. *Nutr Hosp* 2006;21:552-555.

19. Wanke, C.A., et al. A medium chain triglyceride-based diet in patients with HIV and chronic diarrhea reduces diarrhea and malabsorption: a prospective, controlled trial. *Nutrition* 1996;12:766-771.

20. Thormar, H., et al. Hydrogels containing monocaprin have potent microbicidal activities against sexually transmitted viruses and bacteria in vitro. *Sex Transm Infect* 1999;75(3):181-185.

21. Kabara, J.J. *The Pharmacological Effect of Lipids.* Champaign, IL: The American Oil Chemists' Society, 1978.

22. Fife, B. *The Coconut Oil Miracle.* New York, NY: Avery, 2004.

23. http://www.coconutresearchcenter.org/hwnl_5-5.htm.

24. http://www.coconutresearchcenter.com/article10526.pdf.

25. Gordon, S. Coconut oil may help fight childhood pneumonia. *US News and World Report*, Oct 30, 2008.

26. Ogbolu, D.O. In vitro antimicrobial properties of coconut oil on Candida species in Ibadan, Nigeria. *J Med Food* 2007;10:384-387.

182

27. Kitahara, T., et al. Antimicrobial activity of saturated fatty acids and fatty amines against methicillin-resistant Staphylococcus aureus. *Biol Pharm Bull* 2004;27:1321-1326.
28. Ogbolu, D.O. In vitro antimicrobial properties of coconut oil on Candida species in Ibadan, Nigeria. *J Med Food* 2007;10:384-387.

Chapter 7: The Anti-Arthritis Diet

1. Ford, N.D. *How to Eat Away Arthritis and Gout*. Parker Pub Co;West Nyack, NY,1982.
2. McKay, L., et al. Effect of a topical herbal cream on the pain and stiffness of osteoarthritis: a randomized double-blind, placebo-controlled clinical trial. *J Cllin Rheumatol* 2003;9:164-169.
3. Buchanan, H.M., et al. Is diet important in rheumatoid arthritis? *Br J Rheumatol* 1991;30:125-134.
4. Skoldstam, L. and Magnusson, K.E. Fasting, intestinal permeability, and rheumatoid arthritis. *Rheum Dis Clin North Am* 1991;17:363-371.
5. Branch-Mays, G.L., et al. The effects of a calorie-reduced diet on periodontal inflammation and disease in a non-human primate model. *J Periodontal* 2008;79:1184-1191.
6. Kjeldsen-Kragh, J., et al. Controlled trial of fasting and one-year vegetarian diet in rheumatoid arthritis. *Lancet* 1991;338:899-902.
7. Kjeldsen_Kragh, J. Rheumatoid arthritis treated with vegetarian diets. *Am J Clin Nutr* 1999;70:594S-600S.
8. Cleave, T.L. *The Saccharine Disease*. Bristol: John Wright & Sons, 1974.
9. Wang, Y., et al. Effect of fatty acids on bone marrow lesions and knee cartilage in healthy, middle-aged subjects without clinical knee osteoarthritis. *Osteoarthritis and Cartilage* 2008;16:579-583.
10. Cheng, T.T., et al. Elevated serum homocysteine levels for gouty patients. *Clin Rheumatol* 2005;24:103-106.
11. Jonas, W.B., et al. The effect of niacinamide on osteoarthritis: a pilot study. *Inflamm Res* 1996;45:330-334.
12. Wilhelmi, G. Potential influence of nutrition with supplements on healthy and arthritic joints. II. Nutritional quantity, supplements, contamination. *Z Rheumatol* 1993;52:191-200.
13.Travers, R.L. and Rennie, G.C. Clinical trial—boron and arthritis. The results of a double-blind pilot study. *Townsend Letter for Doctors* 1990;6:360-366.
14. Situnayake, R.D., et al Chain braking antioxidant status in rheumatoid arthritis: clinical and laboratory correlates. *Annals of the Rheumatic Diseases* 1991;50:81-86.
15. Kjeldsen-Kragh, J., et al. Inhibition of growth of Proteus mirabilis and Escherichia coli in urine in response to fasting and vegetarian diet. *APMIS* 1995;103:818-822.

16. Anon. Researchers turn fat cells into cartilage. *Science Daily*, March 9, 2001.
17. Prior, I.A., et al. Cholesterol, coconuts and diet in Polynesian atolls—a natural experiment; the Pukapuka and Toklau island studies. *Am J Clin Nutr* 1981;34:1552-1561.

Chapter 8: Rebuilding Damaged Joints

1. Donvanti, A., et al. Therapeutic activity of oral glucosamine sulphate in osteoarthrosis: a placebo-controlled double-blind investigation. *Clinical Therapeutics* 1980;3:266-272.
2. Pujalte,J.M., et al. Double-blind clinical evaluation of oral glucosamine sulphate in the basic treatment of osteoarthrosis. *Current Medical Research and Opinion* 1980;7:110-114.
3. Shankland, W.E. The effects of glucosamine and chondroition sulfate on osteoarthritis of the TMJ: a preliminary report of 50 patients. *Cranio* 1998;16:230-235.
4. National Center for Complimentary and Alternative Medicine. The NIH glucosamine/chondroitin arthritis intervention trial (GAIT). *J Pain Palliat Care Pharmacother* 2008;22:39-43.
5. Donvanti, A., et al. Therapeutic activity of oral glucosamine sulphate in osteoarthrosis: a placebo-controlled double-blind investigation. *Clinical Therapeutics* 1980;3:266-272.
6. Vaz, A.L. Double-blind clinical evaluation of the relative efficacy of ibuprofen and glucosamine sulfate in the management of osteoarthrosis of the knee in out-patients. *Curr Med Res Opin* 1982;8:145-149.
7. Crolle, G and D'este, E. Glucosamine sulfate for the management of arthrosis: a controlled clinical investigation. *Curr Med Res Opin* 1980;7:104-114.
8. Tapadinhas, M.J., et al. Oral glucosamine sulfate in the management of arthrosis: report on a multi-center open investigation in Portugal. *Pharmatherapeutica* 1982;3:157-168.
9. D'Ambrosia, E.D., et al Glucosamine sulphate: a controlled clinical investigation in arthrosis. *Pharmatherapeutica* 1982;2:504-508.
10. Pipitone, V.R. Chondroprotection with chondroitin sulfate. *Drugs in Experimental and Clinical Research* 1991;17:3-7.
11. Vaz, A.L. Double-blind clinical evaluation of the relative efficacy of ibuprofen and glucosamine sulfate in the management of osteoarthrosis of the knee in out-patients. *Curr Med Res Opin* 1982;8:145-149.
12. Crolle, G and D'este, E. Glucosamine sulfate for the management of arthrosis: a controlled clinical investigation. *Curr Med Res Opin* 1980;7:104-114.

13. Deal, C.L. and Moskowitz, R.W. Nutraceuticals as therapeutic agents in osteoarthritis. The role of glucosamine, chondroitin sulfate, and collagen hydrolysate. *Rheum Dis Clin North Am* 1999;25:379-395.

Chapter 9: The Magic of Motion
1. Shih, M., et al. Physical activity in men and women with arthritis National Health Interview Survey, 2002. *Am J Prev Med* 2006;30(5):385-393.
2. Zeller, L. and Sukenik, S. The association between sports activity and knee osteoarthritis. *Harefuah* 2008;147:315-319.
3. Hunter, D.J. and Eckstein, F. Exercise and osteoarthritis. *J Anat* 2009;214:197-207.
4. Penninx, B.W., et al. Physical exercise and the prevention of disability in activities of daily living in older persons with osteoarthritis. *Arch Intern Med* 2001;161(19):2309–2316.
5. Fries, J.F. *Arthritis: A Comprehensive Guide.* Menlo Park, CA: Addison Wesley, 1979.
6. Carter, Albert E., personal communication.
7. Carter, A. *The New Miracles of Rebound Exercise.* Orem, Utah: National Institute of Reboundology and Health, 1988.

Chapter 10: Lighten Your Load
1. Anderson, J.J. and Felson, D.T. Factors associated with osteoarthritis of the knee in the first national Health and Nutrition Examination Survey (HANES I). Evidence for an association with overweight, race, and physical demands of work. *Am J Epidem* 1988;128:179-189.
2. Traut, E.F. and Thrift, C.B. Obesity in arthritis: related factors, dietary factors. *Journal of the American Geriatric Society* 1969;17:710-717.
3. Felson, D.T., et al. Weight loss reduces the risk of symptomatic knee osteoarthritis in women: The Framingham Study. *Annals of Internal Medicine* 1992;116:535-539
4. Christensen, R., et al. Weight loss: the treatment of choice for knee osteoarthritis? A randomized trial. *Osteoarthritis Cartilage* 2005;13:20-27.
5. St. Onge, M. and Jones, P. Physiological effects of medium-chain triglycerides: potential agents in the prevention of obesity. *J. Nutr.* 132;329-332.
6. Lenoir, M., et al. Intense sweetness surpasses cocaine reward. *PLoS ONE*, August 1, 2007.

Chapter 11: Inflammation Busters
1. Srivastava, K.C. and Mustafa, T. Ginger (Zingiber officinale) in rheumatism and musculoskeletal disorders. *Medical Hypotheses* 1992;39:342-348.

185

2. Aggarwal, B.B. and Sung, B. Pharmacological basis for the role of curcumin in chronic diseases: an age-old spice with modern targets. *Trends Pharmacol Sci* 2009;30:85-94.

3. Aggarwal, B.B., et al. Curcumin: the Indian solid gold. *Adv Exp Med Biol* 2007;595:1-75.

4. Funk, J.L., et al. Efficacy and mechanism of action of turmeric supplements in the treatment of experimental arthritis. *Arthritis Rheum* 2006;54:3452-3464.

5. Jagetia, G.C. and Aggarwal, B.B. "Spicing up" of the immune system by curcumin. *J Clin Immunol* 2007;27:19-35.

6. Altman, R.D. and Marcussen, K.C. Effects of a ginger extract on knee pain in patients with osteoarthritis. *Arthritis Rheum* 2001;44:2531-2538.

7. Srivastava, K.C. and Mustafa, T. Ginger (Zingiber officinale) in rheumatism and musculoskeletal disorders. *Medical Hypotheses* 1992;39:342-348.

8. Jacob, R.A., et al. Consumption of cherries lowers plasma urate in healthy women. *J Nutr* 2003;133:1826-1829.

9. He, Y.H., et al. Anti-inflammatory and anti-oxidative effects of cherries on Freund's adjuvant-induced arthritis. *Scand J Rheumatol* 2006;35:356-358.

10. Marcason, W. What is the latest research regarding cherries and the treatment of rheumatoid arthritis? *J Am Diet Assoc* 2007;107:1686.

11. Shukitt-Hale, B., et al. Berry fruit supplementation and the aging brain. *J Agric Food Chem* 2008;56:636-641.

12. Rakhimov, M.R. Anti-inflammatory activity of domestic papain. *Eksp Klin Farmakol* 2001;64:48-49.

13. Lansky, E.P., et al. Ficus spp. (fig): ethnobotany and potential as anticancer and anti-inflammatory agents. *J Ethnopharmacol* 2008;119:195-213.

14. Garrrido, G., et al. In vivo and in vitro anti-inflammatory activity of Mangifera indica L. extract (VIMANG). *Pharmacol Res* 2004;50:143-149.]

15. Tassman, G.C. A double-blind crossover study of a plant protelolytic enzyme in oral surgery. *Journal of Dental Medicine* 1956;20:51-53.

16. Cohen, A. and Goldman, J. bromelain therapy in rheumatoid arthritis. *Penn Med J* 1964;67:27-30.

17. Brien, S., et al. Bromelain as a treatment for osteoarthritis: a review of clinical studies. *Annals of Oncology* 2004;1:251-257.

18. Kim, A.J. and Park, S. Mulberry extract supplements ameliorate the inflammation-related hematological parameters in carrageenan-induced arthritic rats. *J Med Food* 2006;9:431-435.

19. Khanna, D., et al. Natural products as a gold mine for arthritis treatment. *Curr Opin Pharmacol* 2007;7:344-351.

20. Jang, S., et al. Luteolin reduces IL-6 production in microglia by inhibiting JNK phosphorylation and activation of AP-1. *Proc Natl Acad Sci USA* 2008;105:7534-7539.

Index

187

188

Plaque, 71
Plasmodiuim, 36
Pneumonia, 82
Polyarticular juvenile rheumatoid
 arthritis, 18
Polyunsaturated fat, 107-110
Porphyromonas gingivalis, 46
Potatoes, 97
Pregnancy, 64
Price-Pottenger Nutrition
 Foundation, 153
Price, Weston A., 44-46, 56-59, 63-67,
 103-105
Prior, Ian, 100
Processed foods, 162-173
Prostaglandins, 144
Prostatitis, 77
Prosthetic joints, 24, 25-27, 51
Proteus mirabilis, 30-31, 113
Protozoa, 36
Pseudogout, 15-17
Pseudomonas spp., 23
Psoriatic arthritis, 20-21
Pulp, 52, 53
Purine, 15

Quercetin, 150

RBD coconut oil , 141
Reactive arthritis, 19
Real food, 117
Rebounder, 127
Rebound exercise, 127-131, 153
Red palm oil, 164
Renal failure, 62
Reservatrol, 150
Rheumatoid arthritis, 11, 13, 14-15,
 30, 31, 46-47, 113
Risk factors, 109-110
Root canals, 53-66

The Roots of Disease, 61
Rosenstein, Elliot, 47
Rush, Benjamin, 41

Salmonella, 23, 30
Salt, 164
Sargenti paste (N2), 54
Saturated fats, 107-110, 114
Septic arthritis, *see* infectious
 arthritis
Seven-day whole foods challenge,
 115, 162-173
Shingles, 34
Shortening, 107, 109, 164
Silymarin, 150
Skin, 20, 23
Sodium urate, 15, 46, 148
Solanaceae, 96
Spine, 18
Spirochete, 23, 28, 29
Staphylococcus aureus, 23, 61
Staphylococcus, 36
Starch, 105
Stefansson, Vilhjalmur, 100-101
Still's disease (systemic juvenile
 rheumatoid arthritis), 18
Streptococcus, 30, 36, 43
Streptococcus pyogenes, 23, 61
Streptococcus viridans, 23
Stress, 62-64
Sucanat, 164
Sugar, 105-106, 110, 139, 152, 164
Superbugs, 36, 89
Synovial fluid, 10, 11, 24, 30
Synovial membrane, 10, 14
Syphilis, 23, 29, 30
Systemic infection, 152
Systemic juvenile rheumatoid
 arthritis, 18, 32
Systemic lupus erythematosus, 22

191

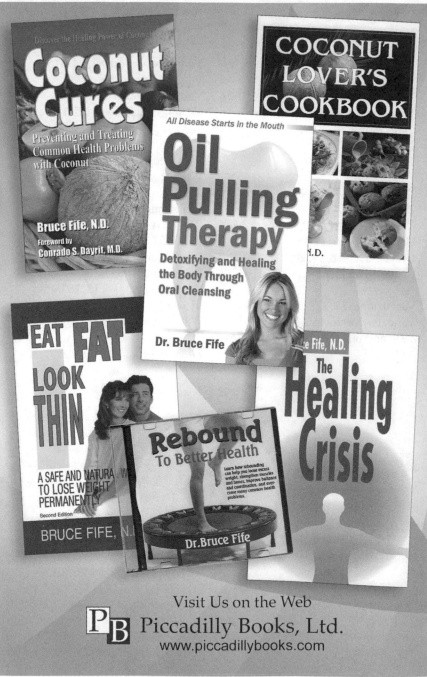

Visit Us on the Web

P B Piccadilly Books, Ltd.

www.piccadillybooks.com